Antigen Absorption by the Gut

Antigen Absorption by the Gut

Edited by

W. A. Hemmings
Agricultural Research Council, Immunology Group,
Zoology Department,
University College of North Wales,
Bangor

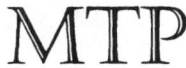

Published by
MTP PRESS LIMITED
Falcon House
Lancaster, England

Copyright ©1978 MTP Press Limited

Softcover reprint of the hardcover 1st edition 1978

ISBN-13: 978-94-011-6611-9   e-ISBN-13: 978-94-011-6609-6

DOI: 10.1007/978-94-011-6609-6

Typeset by Typecrafters Ltd., Preston and printed
by United Printing Services Ltd., Blackpool.

Contents

CONTENTS

List of Contributors

W. D. ALLEN
Department of Immunology, Unilever
Research Laboratory, Colworth House,
Sharnbrook, Bedfordshire

C. ANDRÉ
Research Unit of Digestive
Physiopathology, U. 45 (INSERM),
E. Herriot Hospital, Pavillion H, Lyon,
France

M. R. BRANDON
Department of Experimental Pathology,
John Curtin School of Medical Research,
The Australian National University,
Canberra, 2601, Australia

P. J. BRERETON
Department of Dietetics, Northwick Park
Hospital, Watford Road, Harrow
HA1 3UJ, Middlesex

D. CATTY
Department of Experimental Pathology,
University of Birmingham

A. M. DENHAM
Division of Immunology, MRC Clinical
Research Centre, Watford Road, Harrow
HA1 3UJ, Middlesex

L. DODDYMEAD
Department of Dietetics, Northwick Park
Hospital, Watford Road, Harrow
HA1 3UJ, Middlesex

F. C. DOHAN
Eastern Pennsylvania Psychiatric Institute,
Philadelphia, Pennsylvania 19129, USA

ANNE FERGUSON
Gastro-intestinal Unit, Western General
Hospital, Edinburgh EH4 2XU

M. C. FOO
School of Microbiology, University of New
South Wales, Australia

D. L. J. FREED
Department of Bacteriology and Virology,
University of Manchester Medical School,
Oxford Road, Manchester M13 9PT

R. GINGLES
Forensic Science Laboratories,
Newtownbreda Road,
Belfast

J. L. GOWANS
MRC Unit of Cellular Immunology, Sir
William Dunne School of Pathology,
Oxford

F. H. Y. GREEN
Department of Pathology, University of
Manchester Medical School, Oxford Road,
Manchester M13 9PT

J. G. HALL
Chester Beatty Research Institute, Institute
of Cancer Research, Clifton Avenue,
Belmont, Sutton, Surrey SM2 5PX

J. J. HANKES
Department of Experimental Pathology,
University of Birmingham

R. V. HEATLEY
University Department of Surgery, Welsh
National School of Medicine, Heath Park,
Cardiff CF4 4XN

LIST OF CONTRIBUTORS

W. A. HEMMINGS
Agricultural Research Council, Department
of Zoology, University College of North
Wales, Bangor LL57 2UW

J. F. HEREMANS
Department of Experimental Medicine,
Institute of Cellular Pathology, Université
Catholique de Louvain, 75 Avenue
Hippocrate, B-1200 Brussels, Belgium

A. J. HUSBAND
Veterinary Research Station, Glenfield,
NSW 2167, Australia

A. K. LASCELLES
Division of Animal Health, C.S.I.R.O.,
Parkville, 3052, Australia

A. LEE
School of Microbiology, University of New
South Wales, Australia

G. LOEWI
Division of Immunology, MRC Clinical
Research Centre, Watford Road, Harrow
HA1 3UJ, Middlesex

B. MORRIS
Department of Zoology, The University of
Nottingham, Nottingham NG7 2RD

R. MORRIS
Department of Zoology,
University of Nottingham,
Nottingham NG7 2RD

I. G. MORRIS
Department of Zoology,
University College of North Wales,
Bangor LL57 2UW

A. L. PATEY
Ministry of Agriculture, Fisheries and
Food, Food Science Division, Colney Lane,
Norwich NR4 7UA

B. K. PELTON
Division of Immunology, MRC Clinical
Research Centre, Watford Road, Harrow
HA1 eUJ, Middlesex

D. K. PETERS
Department of Medicine, Hammersmith

Hospital, Du Cane Road, London
W12 0HS

T. PLATTS-MILLS
Division of Immunology, MRC Clinical
Research Centre, Watford Road, Harrow
HA1 3UJ, Middlesex

P. PORTER
Department of Immunology, Unilever
Research Laboratory, Colworth House,
Shornbrook, Bedfordshire

D. I. PRITCHARD
Department of Experimental Pathology,
University of Birmingham

M. SHINER
Department of Gastroenterology, Central
Middlesex Hospital, Acton Lane, London
N.W. 10

R. SOAN
Department of Dietetics, Northwick Park
Hospital, Watford Road, Harrow
HA1 3UJ, Middlesex

J. M. STARK
University Department of Medical
Microbiology, Welsh National School of
Medicine, Heath Paek, Cardiff CF4 4XN

J. P. VAERMAN
Unit of Experimental Medicine,
International Institute of Cellular and
Molecular Pathology, Université
Catholique de Louvain, 74 Avenue
Hippocrate, B-1200 Brussels, Belgium

E. N. WARDLE
Department of Medicine,
Royal Victoria Infirmary,
Newcastle-upon-Tyne NE1 4LP

E. W. WILLIAMS
Agricultural Research Council, Department
of Zoology, University College of North
Wales, Bangor LL57 2UW

J. WOODLEY
Biochemistry Research Unit,
University of Keele,
Staffs. ST5 5BG

ix

1

Introduction

W. A. HEMMINGS

The concept that proteins can enter cells whole is a difficult one. Yet the model situations whereby this process may be studied have been known and investigated for many years. Those situations arise through the specialization required to transfer immunoglobulins synthesized by the mother to the circulation of the fetus or newborn animal, that is in the transmission of passive immunity to the young. This always entails the protein crossing a continuous cellular barrier, in the placenta or fetal membranes, or in the intestinal epithelium.

The concept is hard to accept in terms of cell biology because it is difficult to envisage a mechanism whereby proteins can pass in quantity a cell membrane which is regulating the entry of solutes. Brambell has put forward an hypothesis of such a mechanism, restating it in 'The transmission of passive immunity from mother to young' in 1970. In 1974, after his death, a symposium was held in Bangor largely on this subject, published as 'Maternofetal Transmission of Immunoglobulins'. Since then two further meetings have been held on gut transfer under the title of the present volume, which is composed of papers drawn from these two meetings.

The present position seems to be that considerable modification of Brambell's hypothesis is proposed. There are two main alternatives in sight. The first suggests that incoming protein is taken up in micropinocytotic coated vesicles (MPCV), very ably described by Rodewald, which are assumed, by virtue of their coat of bristles, not to fuse with lysosomes but to pass through the cytoplasm and discharge their contents at the lateral boundary of the cell. But a most important feature of this transport is that it is selective: it differentiates one protein from another in common solution. It is hard to see how the MPCV concept by itself, could explain selection.

The second concept might be termed the glycocalyx assisted diffusion concept, which is based on the twin observations that homologous and heterologous IgG attaches equally to the cell surface, and that apparently any protein administered to the membrane can be found scattered through the cytosol in molecular distribution. It is suggested by Hemmings and Williams that attachment to the glycocalyx is followed by passage of the unit membrane into the cytosol, and that selection occurs at the stage of leaving the cell by assisted diffusion through the lateral membrane.

Further light on this concept is thrown by the observation that the adult gut permits the free passage of large amounts of large cleavage products of soluble dietary protein. This is novel, but extends the older observations that immunologically significant amounts of native protein are absorbed intact from the diet. The cleavage products are found in the cytosol of tissues throughout the body, suggesting that it is normal for these large entities to pass freely into cells of many tissues. This could again be a process of diffusion assisted by glycocalyx material.

These two hypotheses are both closely based on observation, and they are not mutually exclusive therefore. The abused term 'receptor' enters into both, though whether the definitive receptors are in the glycocalyx or upon the apical cell membrane remains to be determined. At any rate, the present position is exciting and changing rapidly.

2

The receptor hypothesis of protein ingestion

I. G. MORRIS

INTRODUCTION

Brambell (1970) has thoroughly reviewed the investigations carried out up to 1968 on the transmission of passive immunity from mother to young in mammals, and consideration of the results pertaining to the rabbit and rodents enabled the formulation of the Brambell Receptor Hypothesis. Until then, the development of this hypothesis had spanned two decades, the first of which culminated in 1958 with the statement of the hypothesis in its original form (Brambell, Halliday and Morris, 1958). The second decade saw several restatements of the hypothesis in the light of new evidence (Brambell, 1963; Brambell, Hemmings and Morris, 1964; Brambell, 1966), and terminated in 1970 with a full evaluation of the hypothesis (Brambell, 1970). At that time, the originator of the hypothesis believed that it left many questions unanswered and would inevitably have to be modified and adapted to further advances.

THE FIRST DECADE

Throughout this period, relevant work had been conducted in ignorance of the structure and complexity of the immunoglobulins. The antibodies used were classifiable into 7S or 19S proteins, or into electrophoretically slow or fast gamma-globulins, though from the mode of their production or isolation into serum fractions, it is almost certain that they can be retrospectively classified into IgM or IgG classes. At the formulation of the first version of the receptor hypothesis, the knowledge concerning the transmission of antibodies or gamma-globulins from mother to young in the rabbit and rodents had been reviewed by Brambell (1958), to whom reference should be made for the full literature.

In the rabbit, transmission occurred entirely before birth, when the yolk-sac splanchnopleur figured prominently in the transfer fetalwards of maternal antibodies secreted into the uterine lumen. In the rodent, transmission occurred mainly after birth when ingested milk antibodies crossed the intestinal epithelium. It was a common feature of these transmitting membranes that the passage of antibodies across them was a highly selective process. Of the several maternal proteins occurring in the fluids that normally bathed these membranes, or in the antisera that were experimentally exposed to them, the antibodies and gamma-globulins, particularly those of the 7S variety, were transferred preferentially. When heterologous antibodies or gamma-globulins were injected into the uterine lumen of pregnant rabbits, or administered orally to suckling rodents, a more subtle capacity of the transmitting membranes became evident from their apparent abilities to discriminate between the administered proteins according to their species of origin, transmitting some of them better than others. In the rabbit, selection of the protein for transmission to the fetus occurred before its entry into the circulation, and probably within the endodermal cells of the yolk-sac. Entry of protein into these cells was non-selective and was probably effected by pinocytosis. By analogy, it was also considered probable at the time that this would also be true for the absorptive cells of the gut of the suckling rodent.

Another phenomenon pertaining to the transmission of antibodies across the gut of suckling rodents was discovered shortly before the first formulation of the receptor hypothesis, when it was noted that the normal sera of certain species when mixed with an immune serum given orally to young mice or rats, reduced the entry of the antibodies into the circulation relative to similar admixture with homologous serum. This effect, termed interference, could not be attributed to the simple effect of dilution of the antibodies presented to the gut for absorption, since its intensity varied markedly with the species of origin of the interfering sera. The interference capacity of any serum could be reproduced almost entirely by its isolated gamma-globulin fraction, but not by its albumin fraction. Whether the other serum fractions contributed to the effect was

4

obscure, since sufficiently pure preparations of them were not available for testing. Interference had not by that time been observed to occur in connection with the transmission of antibodies across the yolk-sac of the rabbit, possibly because the experimental procedures employed had not been designed to test for it. Nor has anyone since tested for the phenomenon in the rabbit, though more recently it has been shown that the transfer mechanism is a saturable one (Slade, 1969: cited by Wild, 1974) and, on theoretical grounds (see below), should be susceptible to interference.

It was the phenomenon of interference rather than of selective transmission which first suggested the idea of competition of substrate for some kind of receptor. Although selection and interference were both concerned with the transmission of antibodies across membranes and both displayed a high degree of specificity, there did not appear to be a clear relationship between them. Thus, in young rats the homologous antibodies were transmitted much more readily than rabbit antibodies, while sheep antibodies were barely transmitted at all; yet rabbit serum interfered the most with the transmission of rat antibodies, while sheep or rat sera interfered little. On this, and other similar evidence, it appeared at the time that selection and interference were distinct phenomena. Nevertheless, it was considered that the formulation of any transmission hypothesis involving receptors inevitably had to take into account the phenomenon of selective transmission.

Consequently, to account for both phenomena, it was assumed (Brambell et al., 1958) that the absorptive cells of the rabbit yolk-sac and of the suckling rodent intestine possessed receptors adapted to the homologous gamma-globulin, but capable of acting as receptors for heterologous gamma-globulins according to the degree of their resemblance to the homologous gamma-globulin (Figure 1). Common receptors were envisaged, since it was inconceivable that the absorptive cells already possessed specific receptors fortuitously adapted to each type of gamma-globulin which they were capable of transporting, or could produce such receptors de novo. It was believed that the gamma-globulin molecules of several species might resemble each other sufficiently over parts of their surface to effect partial attachment to a common receptor. The degree of resemblance to the homologous gamma-globulin could provide a basis for selection if the probability and/or the duration of attachment of the gamma-globulin molecules to the common receptor were related to goodness of fit. Interference could then be accounted for by the blocking of the receptor-

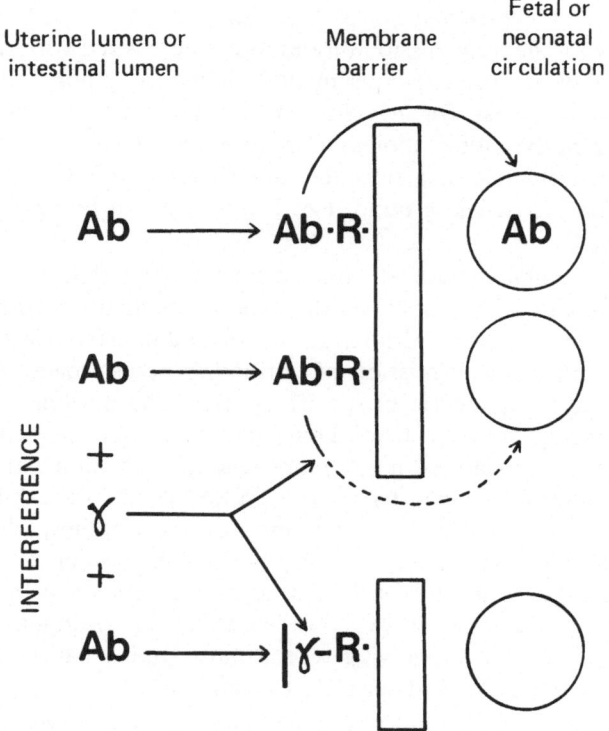

Figure 1 Schematic representation of the original Brambell receptor hypothesis for the transmission of antibodies across fetal or neonatal membranes

substrate system in some way.

At this stage in the development of the receptor hypothesis, there was no indication available for the location of the receptors within or on the absorptive cells, nor of their nature. In ignorance of immunoglobulin structure, it was reasonably considered that attachment to the receptor involved only a short length of the transported gamma-globulin molecule without substantial unfolding and possibly irreversible loss of specific biological activity. Despite such limited attachment, the receptor was considered to be too complex to be as simple as a polypeptide enzyme molecule, otherwise its blockage by interfering protein could not possibly be subject to such subtle specificity. Rather, the receptor envisaged could be likened to a template or mould involved in normal protein synthesis,

6

whether these by RNA or not. It had been realized some time before this formulation of the receptor hypothesis, that the transmission of antibodies across the rabbit yolk-sac or across the suckling rodent intestine was accompanied by marked substrate degradation, but the exact location of degradation was not appreciated, at least in the rodent, until some time later. Association of substrate degradation with the receptor hypothesis occurred in the next decade to account for selection and interference in the presence of substrate degradation, the receptor's main function still being to select and transport substrate, and only secondarily to protect it from degradation.

THE SECOND DECADE

Four main areas of research influenced the elaboration of the receptor hypothesis in its second decade of formulation:

Substrate degradation

Firstly came the realization that the transmission of antibodies and gamma-globulins across the rabbit yolk-sac and across the suckling rodent intestine was accompanied by heavy substrate degradation. In the pregnant rabbit, the fates of rabbit and bovine iodine-131 labelled gamma-globulins injected into the uterine lumen was investigated by Hemmings (1957). Standard concentrations of these proteins were injected into each horn in unilateral pregnancies at doses of 1 ml to each sterile horn, and 1 ml per fetus to each gravid horn. Loss of administered protein through injection punctures or the cervix was prevented by ligatures. The distribution of radioactivity in the conceptuses was determined after 24 h, and the findings are summarized in Table 1.

Degradation of injected protein in the uterine lumen was negligible. Therefore, comparing items 1 and 2, it had to be concluded that the larger proportion of the injected protein had been absorbed from the gravid horn by the conceptuses (item 3), the proportion absorbed being very similar for both rabbit and bovine proteins. Thus absorption was non-selective. However, since only a small proportion of the absorbed protein was recoverable intact in the fetuses (item 4), the proportion being characteristic of the species of origin of the gamma-globulin, and since the fetuses themselves could not discriminate between the bovine and rabbit gamma-globulins in their circulation (Hemmings and Oakley, 1957), the conclusion was inescapable that selection occurred after entry

7

Table 1 Fate of rabbit or bovine iodine-labelled IgG injected into the uterine lumen in 24-days pregnant rabbit. The values recorded are in terms of % of the dose injected

Item	Rabbit	Bovine	Selection
1. % absorbed from sterile horn	24.1		
2. % absorbed from gravid horn	91.3	91.8	−
3. % absorbed by the conceptuses	67.2	67.7	−
% of dose recovered in fetuses			
4. Protein-bound radioactivity	12.1	5.5	+
(a) fixed in carcase	5.0	5.0	−
(b) circulating gamma-globulin	7.1	0.5	+
5. Degradation products (free iodide, after equilibration with the maternal circulation)	18.2	19.8	±
6. % of dose absorbed by the conceptuses, but degraded	55.1	62.2	±

After Hemmings (1957)

of the gamma-globulins into the yolk-sac splanchnopleur but before their appearance in the fetal circulation. The larger proportion of the dose absorbed by the conceptuses but not recoverable in the fetuses (item 6) must have been degraded in the yolk-sac. According to item 5, only slightly more degradation products were recoverable in the fetuses when bovine gamma-globulin was used than when rabbit gamma-globulin was used, but the values recorded are in keeping with the proportions shown in item 6. The values in item 5 were minimum estimates for degradation, since they were obtained after equilibration with the maternal circulation. Comparing items 4 and 6, selection most probably operated as between the proportions of the absorbed gamma-globulins which escape degradation during transmission rather than as between the proportions degraded.

The most likely candidate responsible for the substrate degradation during transmission across the yolk-sac was the lysosomal system of the endodermal absorptive cells. The protease activities of extracts of the yolk-sac splanchnopleur and other fetal membranes and liver were estimated by Jones (1966). Marked activities were found against bovine albumin as substrate at a pH optimum of 3.6 in the yolk-sac, but markedly lower activities in the other tissues tested. From their biophysical properties and substrate specificities, the proteases were found to include cathepsins A, B and C, as well as three other

8

exo-peptidases. Also, cathepsin D was tentatively recognized from its electrophoretic behaviour. The presence of cathepsin D in vesicles within the cytoplasm of the endodermal cells of the rabbit yolk-sac splanchnopleur has more recently been confirmed by Wild (1976). Bovine albumin and gamma-globulin, and rabbit gamma-globulin were degraded by these proteases at pH 5, initially into high molecular weight fragments, and then rapidly into small peptides and amino acids. Although the bovine albumin was broken down more rapidly than either of the gamma-globulins, there was no evidence that the enzymes digested the rabbit and bovine gamma-globulins differently.

A similar situation was found to exist in the case of the suckling rodent, since the amounts of antibodies or gamma-globulins recoverable in the circulation of animals fed with these proteins would account for but a small portion of the doses administered. Brambell and colleagues (Brambell, Halliday and Hemmings, 1961) for instance, found that of a dose of iodine-131 labelled bovine gamma-globulin fed to a 14-day-old rat, only a tenth of it was recoverable intact in the circulation 4 h later, even though 70% of it had been absorbed from the intestine. Thus about 86% of the absorbed dose had been degraded.

Immunoglobulin structure

The second area of research to influence the development of the receptor hypothesis arose from the growing knowledge of the structure and properties of the immunoglobulins. After the initial studies of Porter (1959) and Edelman (1959) on the basic structure of the IgG molecule, great strides were made in the 1960s on the characterization of the immunoglobulins and their biological activities. The control of the latter was invariably attributable to the constant Fc part of the molecules as distinct from the variable Fab parts which were found to be responsible for the antigen combining capacity of the molecules. It was not surprising therefore, that the Fc part was also found to have an indispensable role in the transmission of antibodies across the yolk-sac splanchnopleur in the rabbit and across the young rodent intestine (Figure 2). In the rabbit it was found that the Fc part of the rabbit IgG molecule was transmitted almost as readily as the intact molecule, whereas the remaining Fab fragments were transmitted a tenth as readily. In rodents, the ability of the Fc part of rabbit IgG to interfere with the transmission of other antibodies was significantly greater than that of the intact molecule, even though it was itself transmitted very much less

9

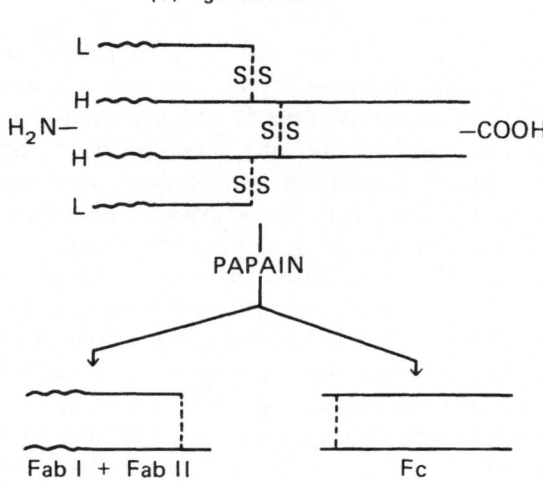

(1) IgG structure

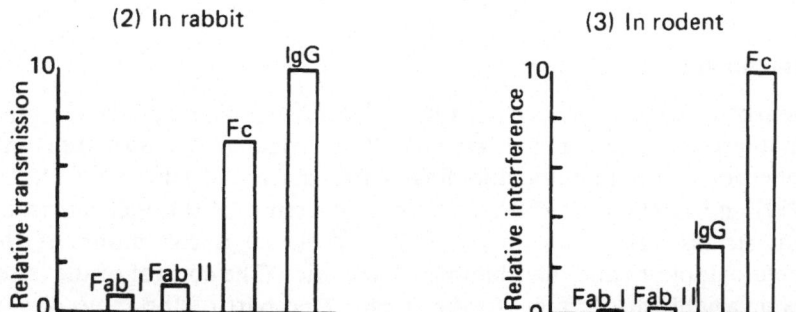

(2) In rabbit   (3) In rodent

Figure 2 The polypeptide structure of rabbit IgG and its papain fragments (1), and their transmission across the yolk-sac splanchnopleur of the 24-days-pregnant rabbit after their injection into the uterine lumen (2), and their capacities to interfere with the transmission of guinea-pig antibodies across the gut of 7-days-old mice, after their introduction into the stomach (3). After Brambell et al. (1960), and Morris (1963)

readily than the intact molecule. The Fab fragments did not interfere to a detectable extent. These observations were most significant, since they made the existence of specific receptors in the recognition stage of transmission much more feasible in the light of the participation of immunoglobulins through their Fc portions in other biological phenomena probably involving attachment to receptors.

Selection and interference

The third significant observation which furthered the development of the receptor hypothesis was the realization that in the rodent selective transmission of antibodies across the gut, and the interference with transmission effected by gamma-globulins, were interrelated effects. It was found that the rate y of transmission of any gamma-globulin across the gut of young mice could best be described by the relationship:

$$y = ax(x+b)^{-1}$$

where x is the oral dose of the gamma-globulin administered, and a and b are constants characteristic of the gamma-globulin (Figure 3). Clearly the constant a is a parameter of selection, since it represents the theoretical maximum transmission of the gamma-globulin at high dosage. Studies on the interfering capacities of several gamma-globulins from different species showed that their b parameters were inversely related to their capacities to interfere and directly related to their susceptibilities to interference from other gamma-globulins. This realization that selection and interference were interrelated effects led to the belief that they were different expressions of a competitive mechanism where substrates competed for a common receptor. The kinetics of such a transfer system are describable by the Langmuir adsorption isotherm (Figure 3). The relationships between a and b, in the above equation, to each other and to selection and interference is exactly the same as the relationships of $K_3 Sn$, and K, of the isotherm, to each other and to rates of transmission and competition for transmission. Thus the experimental results were compatible with theory.

Cytology of absorption

Finally, the other significant advance which led to the furtherance of the receptor hypothesis was the new information from several laboratories about the ultrastructure of the absorptive cells of the rabbit yolk-sac and particularly of the young rodent intestine. Clark (1959) pioneered this field with his studies on the uptake of macromolecules by the gut of suckling rats and mice. Subsequently, several other studies were carried out (reviewed by Morris, 1974) using Evans-blue-protein complexes, saccharated iron oxide, colloidal gold, trypan-blue-protein complexes,

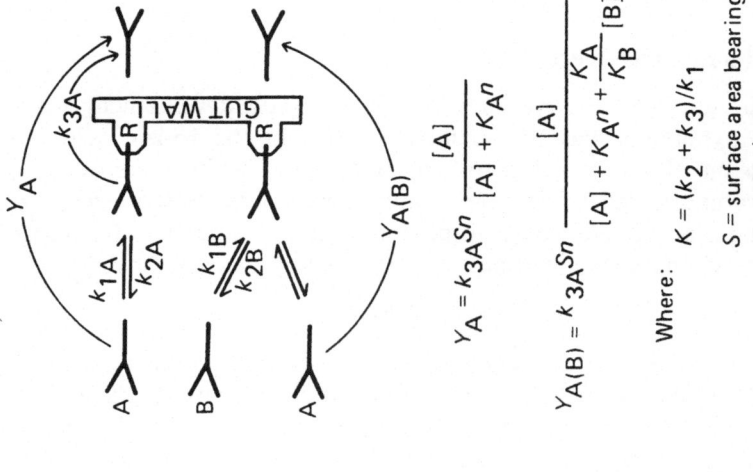

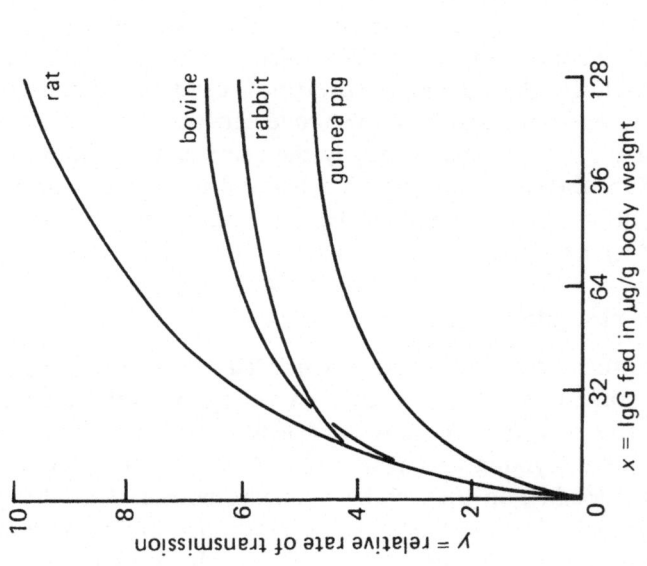

Figure 3 Selective transmission of IgG across the intestine of suckling rodents. After Morris (1964)

ferritin or peroxidase as substrates. Uptake of these substrates into the absorptive cells of the young rodent's gut seemed to be limited to the jejunum and ileum; it was particularly pronounced in the ileum and practically non-existent in the duodenum. In the jejunum and ileum, the free surfaces of the cells are raised into a well developed brush border of microvilli. An extensively anastomosing system of tubules and small vacuoles occupy the region of the terminal web and communicates with the intestinal lumen by occasional caveoli at the bases of the microvilli. Between this system and the nucleus, the cytoplasm is largely occupied by vesicles of varying sizes, mitochondriae and membrane-lined dense bodies considered to be lysosomes. Fusion of some of the larger vesicles with lysosomes convert the former into digestive vesicles. In the ileal cells, some vesicles and dense bodies appear to be discharging their contents into a giant supranuclear vesicle which imparts to the intestine in its distal half a distinctive yellowish-brown colour. After the ingestion of electron-dense substrates, dense particles appear between the microvilli and in the caveoli and apical tubular system at first, and later in the cytoplasmic vesicles and, in the ileal cells, in the giant vesicle. Evidently, absorption into the cell was non-selective. Clark (1959) believed that substrate was absorbed into the cells pinocytotically by the invagination and pinching off of the cell surface membrane at the bases of the microvilli to form vesicles which then moved through the terminal web into the cell. The occurrence in the vesicles of alkaline phosphatase, which is normally associated with the surface membrane, would support this contention. Graney (1968) later showed morphological differences in the unit membrane of different parts of the tubular system and vesicles, and suggested that the apical tubular system and caveoli are a relatively stable system and that entry of macromolecules into them occurs by diffusion. Movement of sequesterd macromolecules thence to the deeper vesicles may occur through the pinching off of small vesicles from the apical tubular system. On the other hand, Vacek (1964) suggested that the vacuolar system represented a certain form of endoplasmic reticulum; conceivably they may represent swellings within the microtubular system. Unfortunately, these investigations employed marker substrates which are not transmitted in significant amounts across the young rodent intestine. Although the results illustrate the uptake of macromolecules into and possibly the fate of macromolecules within the absorptive cells, they furnish no information concerning the exit route of transmitted protein. Less work was done on the rabbit yolk-sac splanchnopleur in the 1960s, though some unpublished studies

13

carried out by W. A. Hemmings at Bangor on ferritin uptake would seem to conform with the type of uptake occurring in the young rodent's jejunal cells.

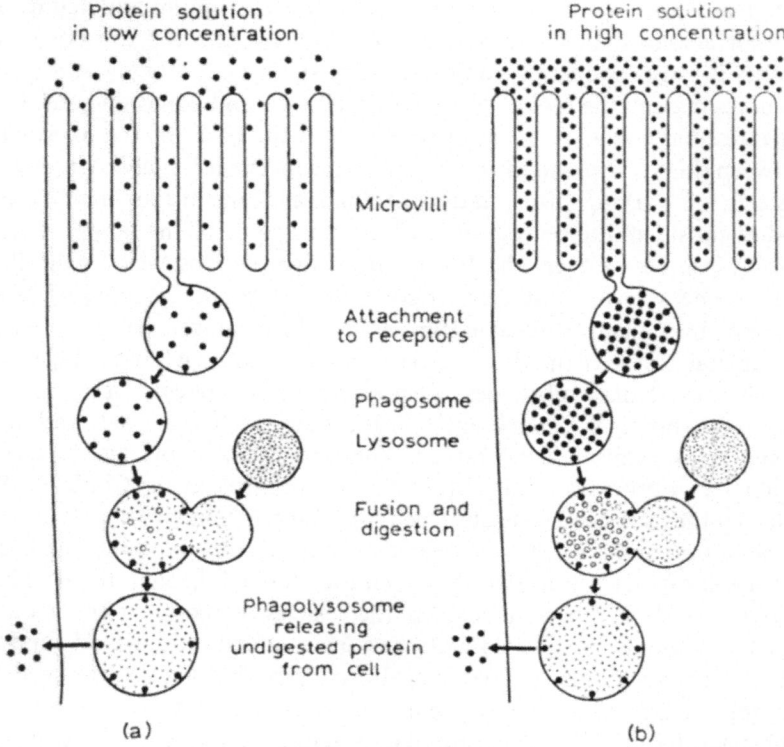

Figure 4 Gamma-globulin transmission across the absorptive cells of the gut of young rodent at low (a) and high (b) substrate concentrations. From Brambell (1966) with permission

In the light of these advances, the receptor hypothesis was restated by its originator (Brambell, 1966), the ultimate form being as illustrated in Figure 4. Common transport receptors were envisaged on the surface of the microvilli, and these were carried into the cell by the invagination of the caveoli so as to become located on the walls of pinocytotic vesicles and phagolysosomes. Entry of substrate into the cells was supposedly non-selective, so that the segregation of transmitted from non-transmitted substrate would occur within the vesicles and phagolysosomes. The receptors were adapted to fit attachment sites found on the Fc portion of the homologous IgG molecules. Similarities to these sites, in

14

the Fc portion of immunoglobulins from other species would enable these proteins also to become attached to the receptors under experimental conditions and to compete for them. Attachment of IgG to the receptors would protect it, whilst substrate remaining free in the phagolysosomes would be degraded. Attached IgG is ultimately released from the cell into the intercellular spaces and thence passes into the lacteals or capillaries. The exact manner of release of transmitted IgG from the cell remained unknown, so that the receptor hypothesis as it then stood did not necessarily imply that all of the phagolysosomal contents including lysosomal enzymes would accompany the transmitted IgG into the intercellular spaces. It must also be emphasised that the prime function of the receptors was to select particular substrates from others for transport across the absorptive cells, and only secondarily to protect the transported substrate from degradation. Over-emphasis on the latter function by several authors has led them to refer to the Brambell receptor hypothesis erroneously as the 'degradation' hypothesis.

RECENT ADVANCES

Some recent advances have confirmed aspects of the receptor hypothesis by providing evidence for the existence of cellular receptors, whilst others have called for yet another restatement of it.

Jones and Waldmann (1972, 1976) have provided convincing biological and biophysical evidence for the existence of receptors in the absorptive cells of the suckling rodent's intestine, which are specific for IgG but not other immunoglobulins. Attachment of IgG to the receptors involved the Fc portion of the molecules and was selective as between the IgG from different species. The receptors are probably located on the microvillus membrane of the cells, since absorption of IgG into the cells as well as its transmission across them was selective. Absorption and transmission were saturable at high IgG concentration, and with a mixture of IgG from different species there was competition for attachment to the receptors. In vitro complexing of IgG with cell membrane material occurred with preparations derived from the proximal third of the small intestine, but not with preparations derived from the distal third. Binding of IgG to cell membrane material was pH dependent, being optimal at pH 4 to 6.5, and reversed at pH 7.4 or above.

Gitlin and Gitlin (1976) did similar work using membrane preparations derived from the cells of young rodent intestine and comparing their results with in vivo transmission experiments. They confirmed that transmission of IgG across the enterocytes involved attachment to cell membrane components, the transmission of different proteins (human IgG and albumin) being directly related to their affinities for the membrane components as estimated in vitro. These authors also confirmed, at high substrate concentration, the saturability of both the transmission mechanism in vivo and attachment to membrane material in vitro. They also showed that individual immunoglobulins in mixtures fed to young rodents competed for transmission in the same order as they competed for attachment to membrane material in vitro. Again the membrane material for study was derived from the proximal half of the small intestine.

In the case of the rabbit, Schlamowitz (1976) investigated the binding of homologous IgG and albumin to the surface membrane of the endodermal cells of the yolk-sac splanchnopleur, and showed that there were specific attachment sites on the membrane for both of these proteins. These receptors apparently constituted distinct saturable transfer systems. The same membrane in the mouse probably performs similar functions as that in the rabbit (Brambell, 1970), and it has been shown convincingly, using the highly specific and sensitive rosetting technique, that receptors are present on the surface of isolated endodermal cells which are capable of binding onto themselves homologous and heterologous IgG molecules through their Fc portions (Elson, Jenkinson and Billington, 1975).

These observations support Brambell's hypothesis as far as the existence of transport receptors is concerned, but they reflect the efficacy of the receptors in controlling the entry of IgG into the absorptive cells, so that selection appears to be an extracellular event. The rodent work also implies that the receptors are concentrated mainly in cells of the proximal region of the small intestine where the lysosomal system is the least well developed. Confirmation of this possibility comes from the observations of Rodewald (1970), Mackenzie (1972), Jones (1976) and the Morris's (1976) that the transintestinal passage of IgG injected into segments of the small intestine of suckling rats isolated by ligatures, is between 10 and 30 times greater in the proximal than in the distal part. Some of these authors (Morris and Morris, 1976) go as far as to claim that the distal part is not transmissible to intact IgG at all. Jones (1974) however, carried out in vitro transmission experiments with sacs of everted intestine prepared from the proximal and distal regions of the

16

young rat gut. Whereas the proximal sacs transferred IgG across their walls the more efficiently, the distal sacs also transmitted to a significant degree. That transport can occur in the ileal region has also been demonstrated by the in vitro experiments of Bamford (1966), showing that this part of the young rodent's intestine can transmit IgG or antibodies intact across its wall in as selective a manner as in the in vivo situation. The involvement of lysosomes (ileum) in the transmission mechanism is strongly supported by the observation made by Halliday (1959) that the intestinal transmission of antibodies in fed rats is doubled when cortisone acetate is administered simultaneously by mouth or parenterally; it is known that cortisone and its analogues stabilize the membranes of lysosomes and prevents them from forming phagolysosomes with pinocytotic vesicles (Weissman, 1968).

The concensus of opinion deriving from these observations is that the proximal small intestine of the suckling rodent is by far the more transmissive region of the gut for IgG, though the distal region may be the more absorptive. It would appear that normally the proximal region selects from the lumen the substrate for transmission into the circulation, mainly the IgG of suckled milk, allowing the remaining constituents to pass into the distal region for absorption and intracellular digestion mainly, though some transmission can also occur here.

Cytological evidence to support the transmission of IgG across proximal intestinal cells of suckling rats, without the involvement of lysosomes, is provided by the work of Rodewald (1973, 1976). Wild (1976) describes a similar mechanism in the endoderm cells of the rabbit yolk-sac splanchnopleur. Both of these authors independently came to very similar conclusions, believing that IgG destined for transport across absorptive cells is first taken into micropinocytotic vesicles selectively, probably through attachment to specific receptors located on the glycocalyx of the apical cell surface, so that it is segregated from non-transmitted substrates before entry into the cells (Figure 5). The transport of such interiorized IgG across the cells differs in the rabbit yolk-sac and rat intestine, but in both it involves movement of IgG-containing coated vesicles which escape fusion with lysosomes. The vesicles empty their contents by reverse pinocytosis at the base of the cells in rabbit or laterally into the intercellular spaces in the rat. Rodewald (1976) also provided evidence supporting that of Jones and Waldmann (1972) that attachment of IgG to the receptors is pH dependent. When IgG buffered to pH 7.4 or 6.5 was infused into the duodenum of suckling rats, its uptake into the enterocytes, observed histo-

17

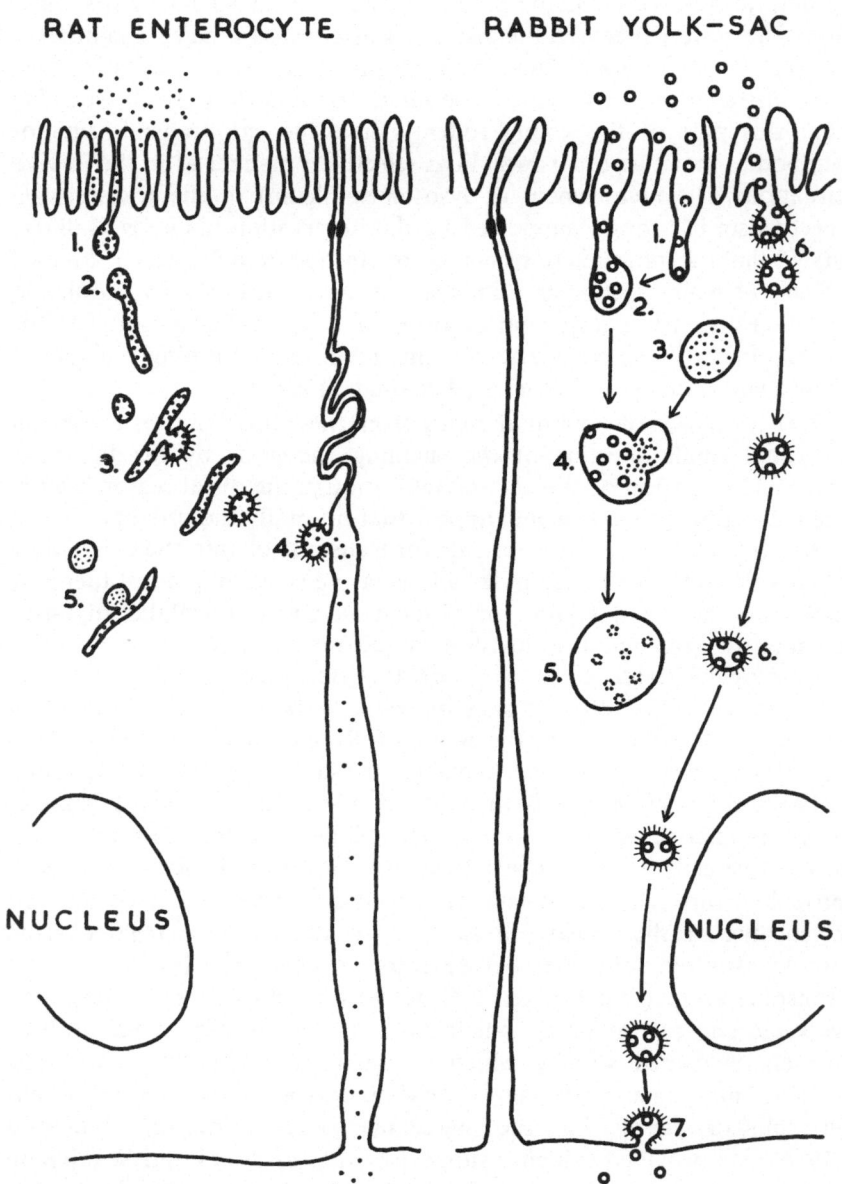

RAT ENTEROCYTE   RABBIT YOLK-SAC

NUCLEUS   NUCLEUS

Figure 5 Routes of transmission of antibodies across absorptive cells of the young rat duodenum and of the rabbit yolk-sac splanchnopleur. In the rat: 1 = selection of IgG by receptors on the walls of small pits

18

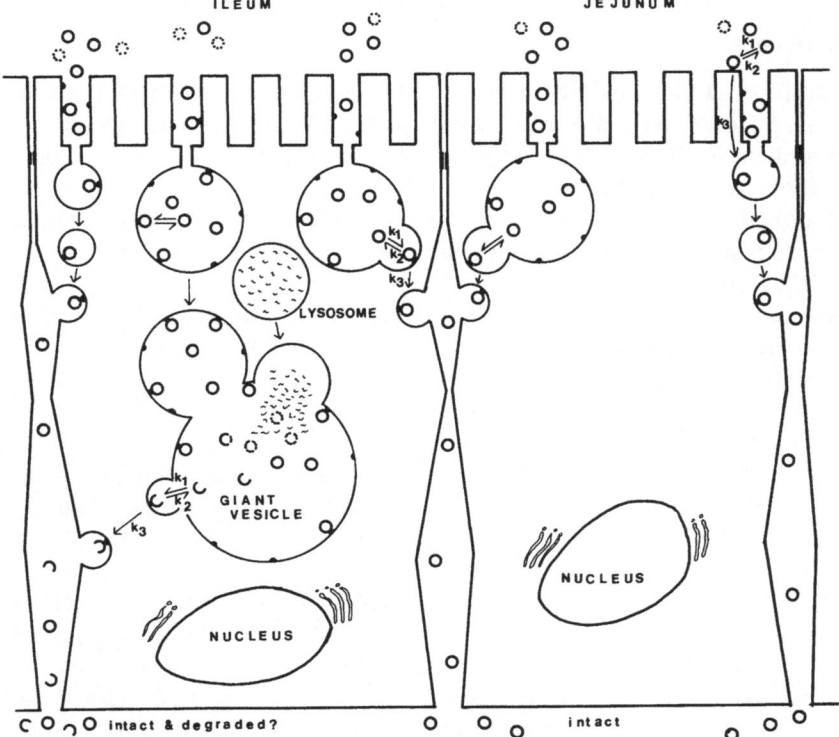

Figure 6 Restatement of the Brambell receptor hypothesis in the light of recent advances

logically, varied inversely with the pH.

In the light of these recent advances, the receptor hypothesis clearly needs a further restatement, and an attempt at this with reference to the young rodent intestine is made in Figure 6. The modifications are readily apparent from the figure and need no further elaboration. Wherever the segregation of transmitted from non-transmitted substrate occurs, it is probably effected by selective receptor-mediated surface endocytosis.

---

forming at the bases of the micro-villi; 2 = pinocytosis and segregation of IgG into tubular vesicles; 3 = transfer of IgG into coated micro-vesicles; 4 = reverse pinocytosis releasing IgG into intercellular spaces; 5 = degradation of excess substrate. In the rabbit: 1 = apical tubules; 2 = pinocytosis; 3 = lysosome; 4 = phagolysosome; 5 = complete degradation of absorbed IgG; 6 = coated micro-pinocytotic vesicle with specific receptors; 7 = reverse pinocytosis and release of IgG into the vitelline circulation. After Rodewald (1973), and Wild (1976)

19

References

Bamford, D. R. (1966). Studies in vitro of the passage of serum proteins across the intestinal wall of young rats. Proc. R. Soc. B, **166**, 30

Brambell, F. W. R. (1958). The passive immunity of the young mammal. Biol. Rev., **33**, 488

Brambell, F. W. R. (1963). Resemblances between passive anaphylactic sensitization and transmission of passive immunity. Nature, Lond., **199**, 1164

Brambell, F. W. R. (1966). The transmission of immunity from mother to young and the catabolism of immunoglobulins. Lancet, **ii**, 1087

Brambell, F. W. R. (1970). The transmission of passive immunity from mother to young. Frontiers of Biology, Vol. 18. (Amsterdam: North Holland)

Brambell, F. W. R., Halliday, R. and Hemmings, W. A. (1961). Changes in iodine-131 labelled immune bovine gamma-globulin during transmission to the circulation after oral administration to the young rat. Proc. R. Soc. B, **153**, 477

Brambell, F. W. R., Halliday, R. and Morris, I. G. (1958). Interference by human and bovine serum protein fractions with the absorption of antibodies by suckling rats and mice. Proc. R. Soc. B, **149**, 1

Brambell, F. W. R., Hemmings, W. A. and Morris, I. G. (1964). A theoretical model of gamma-globulin catabolism. Nature, Lond., **203**, 1352

Brambell, F. W. R., Hemmings, W. A., Oakley, C. L. and Porter, R. R. (1960). The relative transmission of the fractions of papain hydrolysed homologous gamma-globulin from the uterine cavity to the foetal circulation in the rabbit. Proc. Roy. Soc. B, **151**, 478

Clark, S. L. (1959). The ingestion of proteins and colloidal materials by columnar absorptive cells of the small intestine in suckling rats and mice. J. Biophys. Biochem. Cytol., **5**, 41

Edelman, G. M. (1959). Dissociation of gamma-globulin. J. Am. Chem. Soc., **81**, 3155

Elson, J., Jenkinson, E. J. and Billington, W. D. (1975). Fc receptors on mouse placenta and yolk sac cells. Nature, Lond., **255**, 412

Gitlin, J. D. and Gitlin, D. (1976). Protein binding by cell membranes and the selective transfer of proteins from mother to young across tissue barriers. In: (W. A. Hemmings (ed.), Maternofoetal Transmission of Immunoglobulins p.113-119. (London: Cambridge University Press)

Graney, D. O. (1968). The uptake of ferritin by ileal absorptive cells in suckling rats. An electron microscope study. Am. J. Anat., **123**, 227

Halliday, R. (1959). The effect of steroid hormones on the absorption of antibody by the young rat. J. Endocrinol., **18**, 56

Hemmings, W. A. (1957). Protein selection in the yolk-sac splanchnopleur of the rabbit: the total uptake estimated as loss from the uterus. Proc. R. Soc. B, **148**, 76

Hemmings, W. A. and Oakley, C. L. (1957). Protein selection in the yolk-sac splanchnopleur of the rabbit: the fate of globulin injected into the foetal circulation. Proc. R. Soc. B, **146**, 573

Jones, E. A. and Waldmann, T. A. (1972). The mechanism of intestinal uptake and transcellular transport of IgG in the neonatal rat. J. Clin. Invest., **51**, 2916

Jones, R. E. (1966). Studies on the proteolytic enzymes of the foetal yolk sac of the rabbit. M.Sc. Thesis, University of Wales

Jones, R. E. (1974). Studies in vivo and in vitro of the transfer of rat IgG and rat albumen across the intestinal walls of young rats. Biol. Neonat, **24**, 220

Jones, R. E. (1976). Studies on the transmission of bovine IgG across the intestine of the young rat. In: (W. A. Hemmings (ed.), Maternofoetal Transmission of Immunoglobulins p.325—337. (London: Cambridge University Press)

Mackenzie, D. D. S. (1972). Selective uptake of immunoglobulin by the proximal intestine of suckling rats. Am. J. Physiol., **223**, 1286

Morris, B. and Morris, R. (1976). Quantitative assessment of the transmission of labelled protein by the proximal and distal regions of the small intestine of young rats. J. Physiol., **255**, 619

Morris, I. G. (1963). Interference with the uptake of guinea-pig agglutinins in mice due to fractions of papain hydrolysed rabbit gamma-globulin. Proc. R. Soc. B, **157**, 160

Morris, I. G. (1964). The transmission of antibodies and normal gamma-globulins across the young mouse gut. Proc. R. Soc. B, **160**, 276

Morris, I. G. (1974). Immunological proteins. In: (D. H. Smyth (ed), Intestinal Absorption p.483—540. (London: Plenum Press.)

Porter, P.P. (1959). The hydrolysis of rabbit gamma-globulin and antibodies with crystalline papain. Biochem. J., **73**, 119

Rodewald, R. (1970). Selective antibody transport in the proximal small intestine of the neonatal rat. J. Cell Biol., **45**, 635

Rodewald, R. (1973). Intestinal transport of antibodies in the newborn rat. J. Cell Biol., **58**, 189

Rodewald, R. (1976). Intestinal transport of peroxidase-conjugated IgG fragments in the neonatal rat. In: (W. A. Hemmings (ed.), Maternofoetal Transmission of Immunoglobulins p. 137—149. (London: Cambridge University Press)

Schlamowitz, M. (1976). Maternofoetal transmission of protein in the rabbit: transfer in vivo and binding in vitro to the yolk-sac membrane. In: (W. A. Hemmings (ed.), Maternofoetal Transmission of Immunoglobulins p.179—199. (London: University Press)

Vacek, Z. (1964). Submikroskopická a cytochemie epithelu tenkého streva u krysích mlád'at. Cslká Morf., **12**, 292

Waldmann, T. A. and Jones. E. A. (1976). The role of IgG-specific cell surface receptors in IgG transport and catabolism. In: (W. A. Hemmings (ed.), Maternofoetal Transmission of Immunoglobulins p.123—133. (London: Cambridge University Press)

Weissmann, G. (1968). The effects of steroids and drugs on lysosomes. In: (J. T. Dingle and Honor B. Fell, (ed.), Lysosomes in Biology and Pathology p.276—295. (Amsterdam: North Holland)

Wild, A. E. (1974). Protein transport across the placenta. Symp. Soc. Exp. Biol., **28**, 521

Wild, A. E. (1976). Mechanism of protein transport across the rabbit yolk sac endoderm. In: (W. A. Hemmings (ed.), Maternofoetal Transmission of Immunoglobulins p.155—165. (London: University Press)

3

Macromolecular uptake and transport by the small intestine of the suckling rat

B. MORRIS AND R. MORRIS

INTRODUCTION

Many of the investigations into the uptake and transport of macromolecules by the small intestine of the young rat, which were performed during the 1960s, tended to focus attention on the distal region of the gut. Earlier work, dating back to the studies by Clark (1959), suggested that although fat was absorbed by the proximal small intestine of suckling animals, protein was not. More recently, observations based on electron microscopy studies on the morphological and functional gradients in the small intestine (Graney, 1968), supported the earlier suggestion that intact protein was not absorbed by the proximal intestine and that the cells of the jejunum lacked the morphological apparatus necessary for the absorption of intact protein. Some authors have not clearly distinguished between proximal and distal cells (Kraehenbuhl and Campiche, 1969; Orlic and Lev, 1973) and in some studies the regions of the small intestine under investigation have not been clearly defined.

According to the Brambell hypothesis, antibody protein present in the milk would be taken up by pinocytosis and a certain proportion would become attached to specific receptors, adapted for homologous protein. Such binding would protect these molecules from catabolism. Many of the diagrammatic illustrations and descriptions in the literature, appear to relate more to the cells of the ileal region of the gut, rather than to

23

those of the proximal region. Furthermore, studies on macromolecular uptake, using iodine-125 labelled polyvinyl pyrrolidone (PVP) directed attention towards the terminal region of the small intestine (Clarke and Hardy, 1969a, b). The cells of the terminal ileum took up PVP readily, and accumulated it in their large supranuclear vacuoles, whereas the enterocytes of the proximal region of the small intestine did not take up PVP. The cessation of PVP uptake was clearly associated with the replacement of the vacuolated cells by a new cell type, which was unable to take up PVP. This cell replacement occurred at 18-21 days and coincided with the loss of the ability of the gut to transmit antibody to the circulation (Halliday, 1955). It has been shown that treatment with certain steroids led to a precocious replacement of the cells of the distal small intestine and to the loss of the ability to take up PVP (Daniels et al., 1973); this treatment also caused precocious termination of antibody transmission (Halliday, 1959; Jones, 1972; Morris and Morris, 1974a).

Work which has been performed in recent years has led to a clarification of many of the important features of the physiology of the small intestine of the suckling rat. Morris and Begley (1970) reported the absorption of antibody by the proximal small intestine and Rodewald (1973) suggested, based on his EM studies, that it was the enterocytes of the proximal small intestine that selectively transported antibody to the circulation and that the cells of the distal region digested proteins non-selectively. The transmission of homologous, labelled IgG by the proximal small intestine and the failure of the ileum to do so, has been clearly demonstrated (Morris and Morris, 1974b, 1975; Morris, 1975) and the work of Jones and Waldmann (1972) has provided proof of the complexing of IgG to receptors in homogenates of proximal enterocytes but not in homogenates of the ileal region.

In this brief review paper we wish to consider the significance of recent findings to our understanding of some aspects of the physiology of different regions of the small intestine of the suckling rat and to outline certain outstanding problems.

UPTAKE/TRANSMISSION OF LABELLED, HOMOLOGOUS IgG

Concentration quotients (CQ) have been widely used for studying protein transmission by the small intestine. Though acceptable in many circumstances, CQs can only serve as estimates of the amount of protein present in the circulation and give no information about the protein which has left the vascular compartment and passed into other tissues.

In recent studies we measured the plasma volume of 15-16-day-old rats, by injecting iodine-125 labelled IgG into the heart. The rate of loss of IgG from the vascular compartment was assessed and the distribution of radioactivity in the homogenized tissues was measured. These experiments, the details of which are published elsewhere (Morris and Morris, 1976a), showed that labelled IgG left the vascular compartment at the rate of 9-10%/h and that about 11% of the labelled dose was catabolized in 2 h.

In further experiments labelled IgG was injected into the proximal small intestine or into the ileum and the amount and distribution of transmitted, labelled protein was assessed. About half of the injected IgG

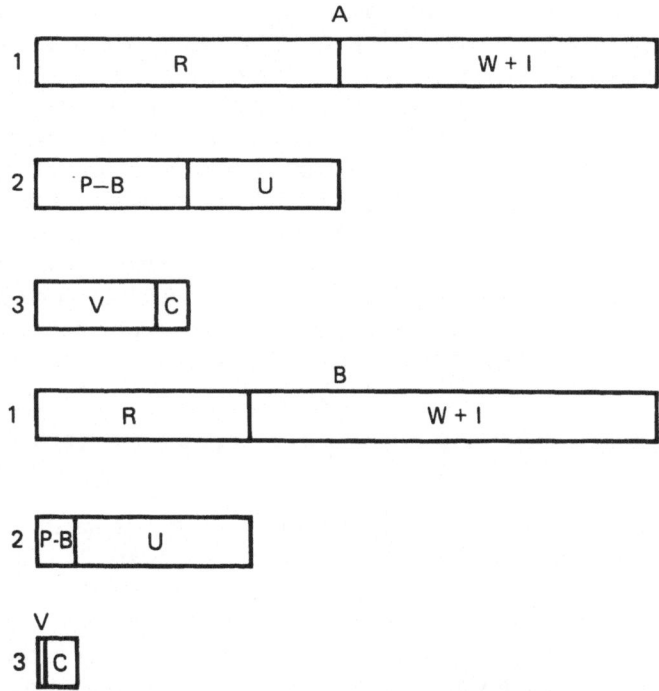

Figure 1 Absorption and transmission of labelled IgG from the proximal small intestine (A) and the ileum (B). 1 — represents the 1000 μg dose injected and shows the amount which has left the intestine (R) and the amount in the gut wash and intestinal wall (W + I). 2 — the amount of protein-bound (P-B) and unbound activity (U) recovered in homogenates of the whole body. 3 — the amount of protein-bound radioactivity in the vascular compartment (V) and that which has left the vascular space (C).

left the proximal small intestine in 2 h and 44% of this was recovered in the body as protein-bound activity (Figure 1a). The rate at which this TCA precipitable, transmitted protein left the vascular compartment (9-10%/h) was the same as that obtained when IgG was injected into the heart — suggesting that all of this transmitted protein was intact IgG. Thus it appears that over 40% of the labelled IgG presented to the proximal enterocytes, without having passed through the stomach, was transmitted intact.

In contrast, after injection into the ileum, only about 16% of the radioactivity which left the intestine was recovered as TCA precipitable protein-bound activity (Figure 1b). Of this about 90% had left the vascular compartment, and only a trace of TCA precipitable activity remained in the vascular space. Thus the TCA precipitable break-down products, and the smaller break-down products which result from passage through the ileal cells, were voided from the circulation very quickly. It is very unlikely that any of this material was intact IgG.

Our results suggested that large molecular weight fragments were not produced during passage through the proximal enterocytes, otherwise the rate of removal from the circulation of TCA precipitable protein-bound radioactivity would have been much faster than that obtained after the injection of labelled IgG into the heart. This may indicate that the passage of IgG through proximal cells may be an all-or-none process. Attachment to receptors may afford complete protection and antibodies which are not so attached may be degraded to TCA soluble fragments.

THE APPEARANCE OF NEW CELL TYPES IN THE SMALL INTESTINE

Continuous cell replacement occurs on the villi of the small intestine; cells arise from the crypts of Lieberkühn and old cells are sloughed off at the apices of the villi. The proximal enterocytes lose their ability to transmit IgG between 18-21 days — a highly significant change in function. Concurrently a new cell type makes its appearance in the ileum, a change which is readily discernible at the light microscope level and was thought to be related to the loss of the ability to transmit antibody. However, this is clearly not so (Morris and Morris, 1974, 1976b; Morris, 1975) and the true functional significance of this change remains to be resolved.

Considerable work has been done to explore the possible underlying causes which trigger the production of new cell types in the small intestine of 18-21-day-old rats, but little significant progress has been made. It has been suggested that the adrenal cortex may be implicated in the maturation changes which occur in the small intestine at this time (Halliday, 1959; Daniels, Hardy and Malinowska, 1973). Hardy and his collaborators examined steroid plasma levels during the time of normal closure. They showed that corticosterone levels tended to increase after 16 days and increased twofold at 18-19 days. Cortisone is very effective in precociously inducing those changes which occur at the time of closure — cessation of immunoglobulin transmission and the displacement of the vacuolated cells in the ileum. However, cortisone is not present in rats in significant amounts under normal conditions and corticosterone is the main adrenal steroid in the rat. We have shown that corticosterone produced some reduction in the transmission of labelled IgG, 3 days after injection into 12-day-old rats, but 4 and 5 days after injection the reduction was less marked and transport function was being re-established (Morris and Morris, 1976a). The uptake of PVP by the ileum, from doses injected into it, was unaffected by corticosterone treatment. Corticosterone treatment did not lead to the precocious appearance of a new cell type in the ileum, whereas cortisone induced this change and led to a drastic cut in PVP uptake.

An examination of the timing of these induces changes is worthwhile. Cortisone, administered at 12 days, led to an almost complete replacement of the ileal vacuolated cells in 3-3½ days. In some of our material the apices of the ileal villi still contained vacuolated cells 3½ days after treatment. Reduction in PVP uptake to the 22 day level (Morris and Morris, 1976a) was dependent upon the complete removal of the vacuolated cells. However, the effects of cortisone on the proximal intestine were achieved much more rapidly. Significant reduction of transmission of labelled IgG, as judged by CQs, occurred after 24 h (Morris and Morris, 1974a) and complete closure occurred after about 48 h (Halliday, 1959; Jones, 1971; Morris and Morris, 1974a). It is very improbable that complete cell replacement could take place at this rate, so much more quickly than it occurs in the ileum. It is more probable that cortisone and corticosterone may repress the function and/or the synthesis of the IgG receptors of the enterocytes of the proximal small intestine.

27

ACKNOWLEDGEMENT

The authors are grateful to the Medical Research Council for financial support.

References

Clark, S. L. (1959). The ingestion of proteins and colloidal materials by columnar cells of the small intestine of suckling rats and mice. J. Biophys. Biochem. Cytol., **5**, 41

Clarke, R. M. and Hardy, R. N. (1969a). The use of polyvinyl pyrrolidone (K60) in the quantitative assessment of the uptake of macromolecular substances by the intestine of the young rat. J. Physiol., **204**, 113

Clarke, R. M. and Hardy, R. N. (1969b). An analysis of the mechanism of uptake of macromolecular substances by the intestine of the young rat (closure). J. Physiol., **204**, 127

Daniels, V. G., Hardy, R. N. and Malinowska, K. W. (1973). The effect of adrenalectomy or pharmacological inhibition of adrenocortical function on macromolecular uptake by the newborn rat intestine. J. Physiol., **229**, 697

Daniels, V. G., Hardy, R. N., Malinowska, K. W. and Nathanielz, P. W. (1973). The influence of exogenous steroids on macromolecular uptake by the small intestine of the new born rat. J. Physiol., **229**, 681

Graney, D. O. (1968). The uptake of ferritin by ileal absorptive cells in suckling rats. An electron microscope study. Am. J. Anat., **123**, 227

Halliday, R. (1955). The absorption of antibodies from immune sera by the gut of the young rat. Proc. R. Soc. B, **143**, 408

Halliday, R. (1959). The effect of steroid hormones on the absorption of antibodies by the young rat. J. Endocrinol., **18, 56**

Jones, E. A. and Waldmann, T. A. (1972). The mechanism of intestinal uptake and transcellular transport of IgG in the neonatal rat. J. Clin. Invest., **51**, 2916

Jones, R. E. (1972). Intestinal absorption and gastro-intestinal digestion of protein in young rats during the normal and cortisone-induced post-closure period. Biochim. Biophys. Acta, **274**, 412

Kraehenbühl, J. P. and Campiche, M. A. (1969). Early stages of intestinal absorption of specific antibodies in the newborn. An ultrastructural, cytochemical and immunological study in pig, rat and rabbit. J. Cell. Biol., **42**, 345

Morris, B. (1975). The transmission of iodine-125 labelled immuno-globulin G by proximal and distal regions of small intestine of 16-day-old rats. J. Physiol., **245**, 249

Morris, B. and Begley, D. J. (1970). The absorption of antibody by the duodenum and jejunum in young rats. J. Zool. Lond., **162**, 453

Morris, B. and Morris, R. (1974a). The effects of cortisone acetate on stomach evacuation and the absorption of iodine-125 labelled globulins in young rats. J. Physiol., **240**, 79

Morris, B. and Morris, R. (1974b). The absorption of iodine-125 labelled immunoglobulin G by different regions of the gut in young rats. J. Physiol., **241**, 761

Morris, B. and Morris, R. (1975). Globulin transmission by the gut in young rats, and the effects of cortisone acetate. In: Maternofoetal Transmission of Immunoglobulins, pp.359-369. (Cambridge University Press)

Morris, B. and Morris, R. (1976a). The effects of corticosterone and cortisone on the transmission of IgG and the uptake of polyvinyl pyrrolidone by the small intestine in young rats. J. Physiol., **254**, 389

Morris, B. and Morris, R. (1976b). Quantitative assessment of the transmission of labelled protein by the proximal and distal regions of the small intestine of young rats. J. Physiol., **255**, 619

Orlic, D. and Lev, R. (1973). Fetal rat intestinal absorption of horseradish peroxidase from swallowed amniotic fluid. J. Cell. Biol., **56**, 106

Rodewald, R. (1973). Intestinal transport of antibodies in the new born rat. J. Cell. Biol., **58**, 189

POSTSCRIPT

In recent fractionation studies involving centrifugation in density gradients (Morris and Morris, 1977a) and ultrafiltration techniques (Morris and Morris, 1977b), the digestion and transmission of IgG and IgG fragments by the proximal and distal regions of the small intestine have been examined. We have shown that:

(a)   Proximal enterocytes transmitted about 39% of the IgG which had been removed from the intestine in intact form. Most of this was retained in the vascular compartment; they degraded up to about 57% of the total removed into fragments less than 1000 mol. wt. and about 4% into intermediate sized fragments.

(b)   Distal enterocytes degraded almost 90% of the IgG processed into fragments less than 1000 mol. wt., about 8% as fragments greater than 100 000 mol. wt.

(c) Fragments, of all sizes, were cleared rapidly from the circulation into the viscera and carcass.

References

Morris, B. and Morris, R. (1977a). Fractionation studies on the absorption of labelled immunoglobulin G by the gut of young rats. J. Physiol., **265,** 429

Morris, B. and Morris, R. (1977b). The digestion and transmission of labelled immunoglobulin G by enterocytes of the proximal and distal regions of the small intestine of young rats. J. Physiol., **273,** 427

4

A preliminary study of the binding of rat and bovine IgG to isolated brushborders from neonatal rat jejunum

R. GINGLES

INTRODUCTION

It has been shown (Jones and Waldman, 1972) that rat IgG binds to isolated neonatal rat brushborders. These workers have also shown that binding is pH dependent, maximal binding occurring at pH 6.5. It is suggested that binding may be the selective process by which preferential transport of IgG from the gut lumen to the serum of the newborn occurs.

The present preliminary studies are concerned with examining the kinetics of binding of rat and bovine IgG to isolated brushborders prepared from neonatal rat jejunum.

MATERIALS AND METHODS

Rats 12 days post-partum were killed by a blow on the head and the small intestine removed. The proximal 2.5 cm and distal half were discarded. The remaining jejunum was everted and brushborders were prepared by the method of Forstner, Sabesin and Isselbacher (1968). In order to obtain enough material brushborders were pooled from 10 rats. The final preparation was suspended in EDTA buffer pH 6.5.

Rat and bovine IgG were labelled with iodine-131 using the method of Rosa et al. (1968). Incubations involved mixing a suspension of brushborders with the appropriate protein solution and maintaining at

37 °C for the experimental time. At the end of this time the incubation mixture was filtered rapidly through a 0.45 μm millipore filter. Filters were dried to constant weight, placed on planchettes and counted directly for beta-radiation using a Nuclear Chicago gas flow counter. The rate of binding (V) was expressed as μmoles protein bound/mg brushborder/min and [S] the substrate concentration was expressed as μmolar.

RESULTS

Binding of both rat and bovine IgG was found to be proportional to time at a protein concentration of 10 μM. The effect of increasing protein concentration was measured for both proteins and is shown in Figure 1.

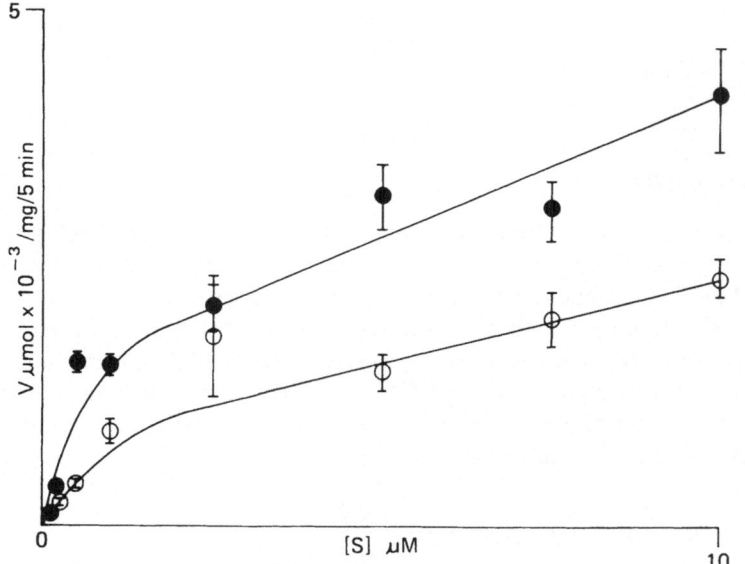

Figure 1 IgG binding as a function of concentration •, Rat IgG; o, bovine IgG

In both cases there is an initial rapid binding rate followed by a decrease in the rate of binding. It would seem that there is a saturable component of binding but at the highest concentrations used there is not complete saturation. The form of the graph may be described by the relationship:

32

$$V = \frac{V_{max} \ [S]}{K_t \ [S]}$$

where V_{max}, the maximum rate of binding and K_t is a constant equivalent to the Michaelis constant of enzyme substrate reactions.

If the data for the saturation curves is plotted using the Hofstee/Woolfe linear transformation the constants V_{max} and K_t may be more accurately determined. Figures 2 and 3

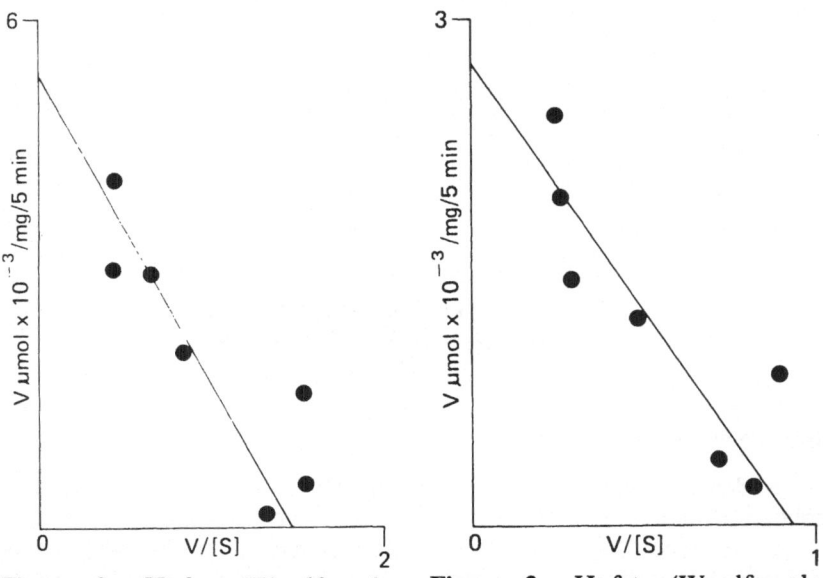

Figure 2 Hofstee/Woolfe plot (rat IgG)

Figure 3 Hofstee/Woolfe plot (bovine IgG)

Rat IgG K = 3.6 μM
Bovine IgG K = 3.1 μM

V_{max} = 5.4 μmoles x 10^3/mg/5 min
Vmax = 2.72 μmoles $\times$ 10^3/mg/5 min

The binding of increasing concentrations of rat protein in presence of bovine protein at fixed concentration 2.5 μM was determined. The results are shown in Figure 4. The V_{max} for rat IgG in presence of bovine IgG is similar to that for rat alone.

Rat IgG in the presence of bovine IgG K_t = 17.33 μM
V_{max} = 5.2 μmol $\times$ 10^3/mg/5 min

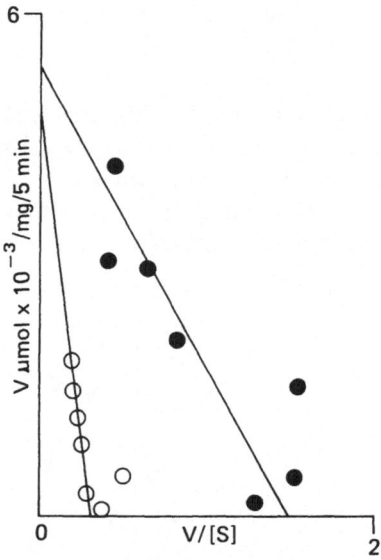

Figure 4 Hofstee/Woolfe plot
•, Rat IgG; o, rat IgG + bovine IgG

DISCUSSION

The evidence presented suggests binding of both rat and bovine IgG to isolated rat jejunal brushborders is at least a partially saturable process. There is evidence that there may be some non-specific binding which may be a property of the brushborder preparation. Further examination of the nature of this non-specific binding will have to be done in order to determine whether it is of significance in the selective protein absorption by the young animal.

The K_t values for both rat and bovine proteins are the same, and there is evidence that they have the same very high affinity for attachment to the brushborder preparation. This supports previous in vivo evidence (Morris, 1957) that bovine IgG interferes with the transmission of rat IgG. The V_{max} value for rat IgG alone and in presence of bovine IgG are similar and this suggests a competitive inhibition of the binding of rat protein by bovine protein.

It is obvious that there is a need for further work to characterize IgG binding, in particular to examine the competitive nature of the process using fixed rat and increasing bovine IgG concentrations. It is also desirable to consider the importance of the non-specific attachment but perhaps such binding studies will give greater insight into the selection of proteins by the neonatal animal.

References

Forstner, G. G., Sabesin, S. M. and Isselbacher, K. J. (1968). Rat intestinal microvillus membranes. Purification and Biochemical characterization. Biochem. J., **106**, 381

Jones, E. A. and Waldmann, T. A. (1972). The mechanism of uptake and transcellular transport of IgG in the neonatal rat. J. Clin. Invest., **51**, 2916

Morris, I. G. (1957). The effect of heterologous sera on the uptake of rabbit antibody from the gut of young mice. Proc. R. Soc. B, **148**, 84

Rosa, U., Scasscellati, G. A., Pennisi, F., Riccioni, N., Giagnoni, P. and Giordoni, R. (1964). Labelling of human fibrinogen with iodine-131 by electrolytic iodination Biochim. Biophys. Acta, **86**, 519

5

The transmission of high molecular weight breakdown products of protein across the gut of suckling and adult rats

W. A. HEMMINGS

That animals could be immunized by oral administration of soluble protein has been known since the turn of the century, when Uhlenhuth (1900) first reported the formation of circulating antibodies by rabbits which had been fed on egg albumin. So far as I am aware this is the first statement of the phenomenon. The subject has since lain in the literature, but seems to have escaped the text-books. There was a good deal of interest apparently in the first decade or two after its discovery, and a number of excellent contributions were made, but on the whole they have been ignored, and their important implications have not taken root, so that the work has seemed to be repeated from decade to decade. But now things seem to be changing. The conference on Coeliac Disease in 1974 may mark a turning point. I should like first to look at the phenomenon in animals, especially the rat, in the hope that we may discover in them models of human pathological processes.

We in Bangor stumbled into this field rather by accident, as I shall relate presently, and when we did I knew only of Winter's work in the 40s, which had interested me as an undergraduate. But I rapidly discovered there was a considerable literature flourishing in the early part of this century. Thus Wells and Osborne (1911) published a substantial work on the oral sensitization of guinea-pigs to a variety of plant proteins. The guinea-pigs could later be shocked by oral doses of the specific protein. It is of considerable historical interest that these authors noted that an animal could not be immunised against a protein which formed a normal part of its diet: this would seem to be a first observation of immune tolerance. People became very busy with such work, and typically in the 20s Hettwer and Kriz (1925) confirmed them, using serum proteins in the guinea-pig, and again in the 30s Ratner and Gruehl (1934) confirmed them again, this time being very careful not to force-feed, so there was no question of dilation damage of the gut. Ratner and Gruehl also very usefully review the literature to that date. Then as I said, in the 40s, Winter was at work in this country, using the Schultze-Dale guinea-pig uterus technique to demonstrate both oral immunization and desensitization: the latter of course requires much more massive passage of immunologically intact protein than is required either to immunize, or shock, so in fact Winter made an important advance, though he himself was much more concerned with somewhat odd thoughts about the nature of the serum proteins.

Now in the 60s Cooper's school were concerned with the passage of antigens from the normal mammalian gut flora, and immunization to these. In the 70s we have two more important schools publishing: in Boston, Warshaw, Walker and Isselbacher have quantitated the uptake of serologically intact bovine albumin (BSA) from the gut of the adult rat into blood and lymph, and they find at least 2% of the dose so taken up. In Belgium and France, Dr. Heremans and his associates have been working on oral immunization, and have even shown it is possible to immunize against red cells by this route. More particularly interesting to us at present is the paper by André, Lambert, Heremans and Bazin (1974) in which they show that a preliminary oral dose of human serum albumin (HSA) fed to adult rats reduces the later transport of a labelled test dose across the gut.

It seems we must accept that it is normal for an animal to be immunised by the protein in its feed, and that there is an immunological screen which must be constantly renewed which prevents these antigens from being distributed through the vascular system after each meal. This screen can go wrong, and then we get the enteropathies in animal and human. There is of course a vast literature on human enteropathies, but I would not venture to discuss it.

Now, we here in Bangor came into this field by a back door. We have a history of interest in gut transmission of proteins, antibody and IgG, in the suckling rat and mouse. Halliday and Morris worked for years under

Rogers Brambell on these topics, and Brambell has summarized their work in his final book (1970). More recently, we have now been looking at the mechanisms of uptake quantitatively and on the E.M. by autoradiography, and we find there are two distinct mechanisms at work in the suckling rat. (Hemmings, 1975a). They overlap of course, but in the duodenum there is a process typical of the transmission of passive immunity, the transfer of whole native protein, with less proteolysis and a greater degree of selectivity between homologous and heterologous IgG. In the ileum there is also a massive transport of protein, but this is found less in the circulation than in the carcase macerate. It is typically high molecular weight breakdown products (BDPs) of the IgG or other protein (Hemmings, 1975b, d.). Thus Table 1 illustrates the uptake of ferritin BDPs to the carcase after injecting iodine labelled material into tied off segments of the gut. As you can see, uptake is greatest from the ileal region. I emphasise that this is uptake measured into the tissues rather than into the circulation . . . the latter is much lower, and as between segments is greatest from the duodenum (Table 2). When the serum is tested with specific antiserum after an ileal injection, Table 3 shows that only one quarter of the protein-bound radio-activity is specifically precipitable: that is, three-quarters of this activity, while still present as tungstic acid precipitable material, has lost its immunological specificity as ferritin. Putting these facts together, we suggest that ferritin passing through especially the ileal region is partially degraded, and the BDPs, no longer reactive with specific antiserum, pass rapidly out of the circulation into the tissues; that is, we predict the BDPs to have a short half life in the circulation.

Table 1 Percentage of the total activity injected present in samples of gut, washings, and carcase three hours after injecting iodine-131-ferritin into isolated segments of young rat small intestine in vivo. Means of five animals

Sample	Duodenum Mean ± SE		Jejunum Mean ± SE		Ileum Mean ± SE	
Gut segment injected	9.30	1.03	21.4	4.31	26.1	4.50
Washing	66.4	2.23	59.2	5.10	37.7	2.94
Carcase	24.3	1.32	19.4	2.40	36.2	5.82

Table 2 Percentage of the total activity injected present in samples of gut, washings, and carcase three hours after injecting iodine-125 rat IgG into isolated segments if young rat small intestine in vivo means of five animals

Sample	Duodenum Mean ± SE		Jejunum Mean ± SE		Ileum Mean ± SE	
Gut segment						
injected	8.6	0.64	15.3	2.66	16.1	2.53
Washings	29.5	2.35	49.9	7.91	26.9	3.05
Carcase	61.9	2.13	34.7	5.30	57.0	2.71

What is the molecular form of these BDPs? Figure 1 gives the scan of a sugar gradient ultracentrifugation run on a carcase macerate preparation following feeding of labelled ferritin. The dotted line gives the distribution of the markers, ferritin, BSA and hog stomach pepsin, labelled with iodine-125, whereas the ferritin fed was labelled with iodine-131. You can see there is practically no 131 activity under the ferritin peak, but very considerable amounts at the level of BSA and even more at the level of pepsin (33 000 Daltons). There is a decline at the top of the tube where the small peptides and amino acids are. So you can see that this evidence suggests the ferritin has been cleaved down to entities of size ranging from 5 to 3S. These are still substantial molecules, and definitely in the range of size to react immunologically, if no longer as antigens against antiferritin antibody, yet still probably capable of acting as immunogens in provoking an immune response in their own right.

This situation holds true for molecules other than ferritin. Table 4 presents the outcome of experiments with iodine-125 — rat IgG, where although the greatest absorption is now in the duodenal region (remember this is the homologous protein) the ileal absorption is very

Table 3 The proportion of the protein-bound radioactivity of young rat serum, following ileal injection of iodine-131 ferritin, which is specifically precipitable using a rat anti-ferritin antiserum

Sample	% Specifically precipitable Mean ± SE	
Young rat serum	25.8	3.5
Injected ferritin (mean of three determinations)	97.7	

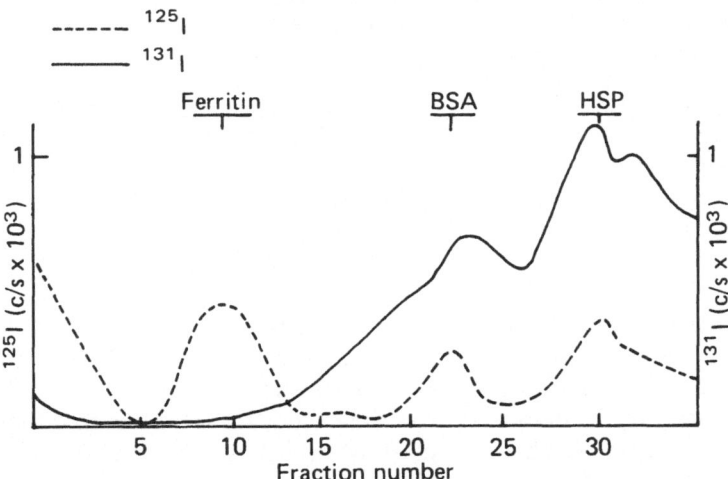

Figure 1 Sugar gradient ultracentrifugation scan of carcase macerate of suckling rats after feeding iodine-131 labelled ferritin. The macerates were spun at 100 0000 g for 15 minutes to clarify, and loaded on 5-40% sucrose gradients, which were centrifuged in the Sw 39 rotor of a Spinco Model L at 39 000 r.p.m. for 18 hours. Iodine-125 labelled markers of ferritin, bovine serum albumin (BSA) and hog stomach pepsin (HSP) were added before spinning

close behind it, in fact probably not significantly different in a large scale experiment. Figure 2 presents the ultracentrifugal scan following feeding of rat IgG. Transfer of passive immunity across the gut ceases sharply at 21 days in the young rat, and this is presumably the closure of the duodenal mechanism. We were lead to wonder if the ileal type mechanism I have been describing, which leads to the transmission of

Table 4 The percentage of the total activity injected present in samples of the washed gut, the washings, and the carcase, 3 hours after injecting iodine-125 labelled rat IgG into isolated segments of the gut of suckling rats. Means of five animals ± SE

Sample	Duodenum		Jejunum		Ileum	
	Mean	SE	Mean	SE	Mean	SE
Washed gut segment	8.6	0.64	15.3	2.66	16.1	2.53
Washings	29.5	2.35	49.9	7.91	26.9	3.05
Carcase	61.9	2.13	34.7	5.30	57.0	2.71

Table 5 Percentage of the absorbed dose which is present in the carcase as tungstic precipitable material at different ages following the injection of labelled ferritin to the ileum

Age post partum (days)	% Dose in carcase, tungstic precipitable Mean ± SE	
15	25.44	3.7
30	48.65	2.23
60	26.23	8.60

high molecular weight BDPs, also closed down at 21 day. Accordingly I tested 30- and 60- day-old rats for transmission of ferritin, and in fact it turns out the transport of BDPs continues unabated into adult life. Table 5 shows the distribution of dose at these ages, and it can be seen that the tungstic acid precipitable content of the carcase is as great at 60 days as it is at 15. At first this finding shattered us, but I cast my mind back to Winter's work, and then went on to discover that there was an ancient and very well annotated literature on oral immunization. We also found that our friends in Belgium were far ahead of us in the field of oral immunization, and that currently work was going on in Boston and Australia. But all this older and new work was concerned, as was our older work, with the transport of immunologically intact or native protein, IgG in our own case, the albumins in that of the Belgian and American workers. But this passage of intact molecules is very limited quantitatively compared with the passage of BDPs which we now have to consider. As you could see from my Figure 1, the amount of intact ferritin is minute compared with the amount of BDPs present in the tissues. So clearly we have a quite new and large-scale phenomenon on our hands, which must have implications not only in the immunology but in the normal ingestion function of the gut.

To illustrate the quantitative aspect, Table 6 presents the data on the distribution of the dose following the injection of labelled ferritin into the ileum of 30- and 60- day-old rats, the washed gut and the carcase protein and non-protein fractions representing the total uptake. At 30 days, over 40% of the dose is present in the carcase as BDPs precipitable as protein. At 60 days the total absorption during the experimental period is much less, and only 5% of the dose is thus present in the carcase. To avoid this difficulty, it seems proper to calculate the proportion present in the carcase as BDPs as a percentage of the absorbed dose, and this figure at 30 days is 49.8%, at 60 days 25.5%,

Table 6 Percentage of the injected dose in various samples from 30 and 60 day old rats following injection of iodine-131 ferritin into the ileum. Means + SE of five animals

Fraction	30 day		60 day	
Washing	10.30	8.9	79.8	4.4
Gut	11.99	2.02	13.1	6.01
Carcase, protein	43.64	2.42	5.3	1.8
Carcase, non-protein	31.92	1.00	2.4	0.34

taking the gut content into account. Calculated solely on carcase content of protein and non-protein activity, the proportions are 57.7% and 68.8% respectively.

When the carcase macerate of an adult rat fed labelled bovine IgG is run on the ultracentrifuge, the scan illustrated in Figure 3 is obtained (Hemmings, 1975d). This is qualitatively very similar to Figures 1 and 2, implying that the derivatives of IgG in the adult rat are similar in properties to those obtained in the suckling. It remains to discuss whether these derivatives are, as they appear, of molecular size 50 000-20 000

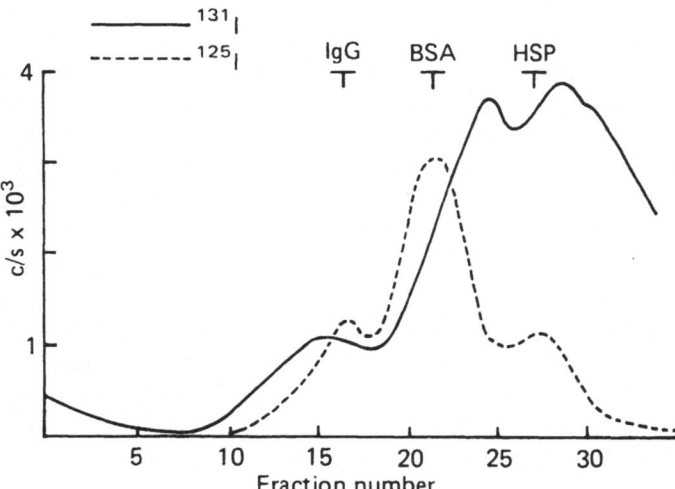

Figure 2 Sugar gradient ultracentrifugation scan of the macerate of the washed small intestine of young rats after feeding iodine-131 labelled bovine IgG. Macerates were clarified as in Figure 1, and loaded on to gradients with labelled markers of bovine IgG, BSA and HSP. They were centrifuged in the Sw 50 rotor at 50 000 rpm for 18 hours.

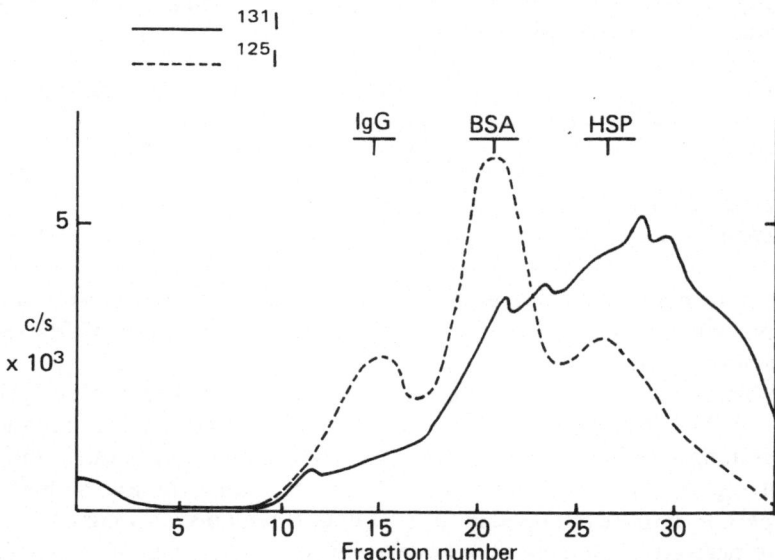

Figure 3 Sugar gradient ultracentrifugation scan of the carcase macerate of adult rats fed bovine IgG labelled with iodine-131. Conditions as in Figure 2

Daltons, or whether these apparent peaks in the centrifuge runs could be an artifact. One possibility is that they represent protein synthesized from amino acid produced by what orthodox teaching predicts as the normal process of luminal digestion in the gut. Many years ago I employed monoiodotyrosine injected into the uterine lumen of 24-day pregnant rabbits to determine whether this amino acid was incorporated into newly synthesized protein in the fetal yolk-sac during transmission to the circulation. These experiments were never published, but gave a uniformly negative result. More recently, Dr. R. E. Jones has carried out similar tests on the suckling rat, and again gets uniformly negative incorporation of amino acid into protein. Iodotyrosine is not a physiologically acceptable molecule for protein synthesis apparently, a most convenient fact when one wishes to use iodine as a tracer for protein.

An even less likely possibility is that small peptides are formed by digestion, and these are being loosely attached to native serum proteins acting as carriers. One argument against this possibility is the relative absence of free small peptides from blood and tissues, as revealed by the ultracentrifuge: this would argue an unusually high attachment coefficient, with the equilibrium far over in favour of the complex. I do not think the physical chemistry of this suggestion is conventional. But the best answer to such suggestions would be the serological one: to pick up the original antigenicity of the molecule in these fragments, thus proving they are larger than merely small peptides. This of course is precisely what Table 3 does in the case of ferritin, for 25% of the protein bound activity of the serum.

This is a very difficult matter to investigate, and in part the problem is enzymological, in part immunological. We are trying a variety of approaches. Mr. Williams is determining the residual antigenicity of the tissues to anti-bovine IgG sera raised in rats, in rats after feeding bovine IgG. He is trying to raise antisera, again in rats, to the natural BDPs of bovine IgG present in rat tissue: if these stimulate antibody formation it would of course be immediate proof of the considerable size of these fragments. But we are also going on to try a variety of other fed proteins: alpha-gliadin, because of its association with coeliac disease, and haemoglobin because of its link with neonatal anaemia. Casein, because of the milk intolerance aetiology, and beta-lactoglobulin, are other possible candidates for study.

References

André, C., Lambert, R., Bazin, H., and Heremans, J. F. (1974). Interference or oral immunization with the intestinal absorption of heterologous albumin. Eur. J. Immunol., **4**, 701

Brambell, F. W. R. (1970). The transmission of passive immunity from mother to young. Frontiers of Biology, In: A. Neuberger and E. L. Tatum eds. Vol 18. (Amsterdam: North Holland Publishing Co.)

Hemmings, W. A. (1975a). Degradation products in gut and carcase tissue after injecting labelled ferritin into the ileum of suckling rats. I.R.C.S. Med Sci., **3**, 216

Hemmings, W. A. (1975b). Degradation products of the Fc fragment of rabbit IgG in young rat gut tissue after injection into the ileum. I.R.C.S. Med Sci., **3**, 280

Hemmings, W. A. (1975c). Transport of protein across the small intestine of adult rats following injection of ferritin to the intestinal lumen. I.R.C.S. Med Sci., **3**, 262

Hemmings, W. A. (1975d). Transport of immunoglobulins across the gut of the adult rat. I.R.C.S. Med Sci., **3**, 282

Hemmings, W. A. and Williams, E. W. (1975). Transport of ferritin across the ileum of suckling rats. I.R.C.S. Med Sci., 3, 215

Hemmings, W. A. and Wood, C. (1975). Selective protein absorption by the gut of the suckling rat following oral immunization. III. Ultracentrifugal analysis. I.R.C.S. Med Sci., 3, 436

Hettwer, J. P., and Kriz, R. A. (1925). Absorption of undigested protein from the alimentary tract as determined by the direct anaphylactic test. Am. J. Physiol., 75, 539

Ratner, B. and Gruehl H. L. (1934). Passage of native proteins through the normal gastro-intestinal wall. J. Clin. Invest., 13, 517

Walker, W. A., Isselbacher, K. J. and Bloch, K. J. (1973). Intestinal uptake of macromolecules II Effect of parenteral immunization. J. Immunol., 111, 221

Wells, H. G. and Osborne, T. B. (1911). The biological reactions of the vegetable proteins I Anaphylaxis. J. Infect. Dis., 8, 66

Winter, L. B. (1944). Anaphylaxis to serum proteins in the guineapig. J. Physiol., 102, 373

POSTSCRIPT

Since the foregoing paper was presented, further work has shown the phenomenon of transport of BDP is present in guinea-pigs (Hemmings, 1977) rabbits (Hemmings, 1977b) and in post-weaning piglets (Hemmings, Kocsis, Pethes and Surjan, 1976). Other proteins have been shown to give rise to BDP, including α-, β- and γ-gliadin of wheat, and mammalian haemoglobin (Hemmings, Patey and Wood, 1977; Hemmings and Williams, 1978).

BDP have been shown to pass other physiological barriers than the gut. Perhaps the most important of these is the blood/brain barrier (Hemmings, 1977c; Hemmings, 1978). BDP also pass the placenta and the mammary gland (Hemmings, 1977d). An hypothesis has been put forward that there is a 'window' for the transmission of BDP of around 50 000 daltons in all cell types. (Hemmings 1978b).

References

Hemmings, C., Hemmings, W. A., Patey, A. L. and Wood, C. (1977). The ingestion of dietary protein as large molecular mass degradation products in adult rats. Proc. R. Soc. B 198, 439

Hemmings, W. A. (1977a). The absorption of iron from oral doses of haemoglobin in adult guinea-pigs. I.R.C.S. Med. Sci., 5, 344

Hemmings, W. A. (1977b). Absorption of bovine IgG by the intestine of the adult rabbit. I.R.C.S. Med. Sci., 5, 286

Hemmings, W. A. (1977c). Dietary protein reaches the brain. J. Orthomol. Psychiat., 6, 309

Hemmings, W. A. (1977d). Transmission of dietary protein across the placenta and through the milk. In O. P. Ghai (ed.) New Developments Pediatric Research pp. 189-192 (New Dehli: Interprint)

Hemmings, W. A. (1978a). The entry into the brain of large molecules derived from dietary protein. Proc. R. Soc B (in press)

Hemmings, W. A. (1978b). Carriage of dietary protein into the tissues. Nature (submitted)

Hemmings, W. A., Kocsis, G., Pethes, G., and Surjan, J. The absorption of iron by piglets from an oral dose of labelled haemoglobin. I.R.C.S. Med. Sci., 4, 392

Hemmings, W. A. and Williams, E. W. (1978). The transport of large break down products of dietary protein through the gut wall. Gut (in press)

6

Ferritin uptake by the gut of the adult rat: an immunological and electronmicroscopic study

E. W. WILLIAMS

INTRODUCTION

The ability of the intestinal mucosa of the adult rat to transmit macromolecules from the lumen to the lymphatics and other organs was studied by means of combined immunological and electronmicroscopic studies of ferritin absorption. After laparotomy and injection of ferritin into the intestinal lumen, small but significant amounts of the protein are transmitted across the gut, probably into the lymphatics, and also to the liver and the spleen. During the experimental period, the intestine retained its normal ultrastructural appearance, and the uptake of ferritin into the cells and intercellular spaces was similar to what had previously been observed in the gut of the suckling rat, when the ferritin molecule was seen to enter the cell and was seen to be present in the cytoplasm, intercellular spaces, and the lacteals.

The small intestine of the adult mammal is not as permeable as that of the neonate, and proteins may be extensively digested by the proteolytic enzymes before absorption by the cells. Data from previous experiments show that the barrier to macromolecules is incomplete, and absorption of amounts of protein from the gut has been demonstrated (Bockman, 1966; Cornell et al., 1971).

In this study, ferritin, an iron containing protein of molecular weight

49

750 000 and molecular diameter, 100 Å was used. Its physiological role is to store iron until it is required for haemoglobin synthesis. This protein is highly electron dense and easily visible under the electronmicroscope. It is also a very good antigen, and can be detected quantitatively by immunological methods, and also vizualized by the electronmicroscope (Williams, 1974).

Previous work on the intestine of the neonatal rat showed that ferritin is taken up non-selectively by the intestinal lining cells by a process of pinocytosis. Within the cell some of the protein is released into the cytoplasm, leaving the cell by a diffusion carrier process through the latero-basal membranes into the lacteals (Williams, 1975). The question that arises from these transmission experiments is whether the protein retains the same configuration after passage through the lumen and the intestinal cells.

The present investigation was undertaken in order to characterize further the extent to which ferritin can be transmitted across the adult rat small intestinal mucosa. These studies include quantitative observations of a preliminary nature by use of immunological methods, and ultrastructural findings on the transmission of ferritin using the electronmicroscope.

MATERIALS AND METHODS

In these investigations, six in vivo experiments were carried out using 260-300 g albino rats of the Wistar strain bred in this laboratory. They were allowed free access to food and water.

Laparotomy was carried out under Nembutal and ether anaesthetic. A midline incision, about 5 cm long was made in the abdomen, and the whole gut gently pulled through to expose the duodenal and ileocaecal end of the ileum, a cut was made at this lower end, and the whole intestine was washed through with 30 ml phosphate buffered saline pH 8 from as near the pyloric end as was possible. This emptied the intestine of all material present, the saline was followed through by an injection of air, which emptied the gut completely. For electronmicroscopic investigations, segments of the duodenum, (1-4 c. caudal to the pylorus) and ileum, (5-8 cm proximal to the caecum) were tied off using Mersilk suture, and a dose of 0.1 ml and 0.2 ml of a 1% cadmium-free extensively dialysed solution of ferritin was injected into these segments, care being taken not to distend the segments and not to leak any of the protein into the peritoneal cavity. For this not to happen, assistance was necessary to tighten the ligatures as the hypodermic needle was withdrawn. After the injections were made, the whole intestine was returned to the abdominal cavity, the animal sutured up and allowed to recover. The animals were killed 3 h later, the intestine was carefully dissected out, the experimental segments separated and washed through with phosphate buffered saline, after which sections of the duodenum and ileum were immediately fixed for electronmicroscopic studies.

Fixatives used were of two kinds:

(1) 1% osmium tetroxide buffered with acetate veronal. (Palade, 1952)

(2) 3% gluteraldehyde in 0.1 sodium cacodylate, pH 7.4 (Pease, 1964).

Table 1 Values obtained from control and experimental tissue homogenate dilutions in agar gel against a rat antiferritin serum

Rat No	Tissue	Control						Experimental					
		0	1	2	3	4	5	0	1	2	3	4	5
1	Liver			+						+			
	Spleen			+					+				
	Serum	−						−					
2	Liver			+							+		
	Spleen		+							+			
	Serum	−						−					
3	Liver	−									+		
	Spleen	−								+			
	Serum	−						−					
4	Liver		+										+
	Spleen		+								+		
	Serum	−						−					
5	Liver			+							+		
	Spleen			+							+		
	Serum	−						−					
6	Liver		+								+		
	Spleen			+							+		
	Serum	−						−					

All tissues fixed in gluteraldehyde were washed overnight in the appropriate buffer, and post-osmicated with 1% osmium for 1 h, prior to washing and dehydration. Osmium-fixed tissue was fixed for 1 h at 4 °C, washed for 1 h with changes of water, dehydrated in solutions of increasing concentrations of ethanol, embedded in Araldite, stored at 60 °C for polymerization. Thin sections were cut on an L.K.B. Ultratome and placed on grids which had previously been coated with an 0.2% formvar solution. A G.E.C. Corinth 275 electronmicroscope was used for all studies.

Preliminary investigations using immunological methods were carried out on the liver, spleen and serum, the results are presented in Table 1 and the immunodiffusion pattern. For these investigations, the organs were macerated in a Tenbrook tissue grinder, using a minimum of saline. Immunodiffusion techniques were carried out in a 1% agar gel medium, (Ouchterlony, 1958). Samples of the macerated tissue were incubated against an antiferritin serum by the radial diffusion method. Control animals used in both studies were rats of the same age and weight, but not subjected to a ferritin injection.

RESULTS

Immunological investigations

After intraluminal administration of ferritin, this protein appeared in the liver and spleen with regularity (see Table 1). In six experiments carried out, these organs of the fed animal contained a higher concentration of ferritin than those of the control animals. There was a rough correlation between the amount of ferritin administered and the amount subsequently found in these organs.

The table presents the data from control and experimental adult rat tissue homogenate, together with serum samples, subjected to radial immunodiffusion in agar gel against a rat antiferritin serum. With the control animals, on average, the liver gives a positive at two dilutions, the spleen at one dilution, with the serum being negative all through.

The data from the experimental homogenate, carried out under identical conditions, against the same rat antiferritin serum are seen to give higher values, the liver gives a positive at four dilutions, the spleen at three dilutions, and again the serum remains negative. The serum in both cases could give a negative result due to a dilution effect.

Figure 1 a and b are immunodiffusion patterns obtained by reacting

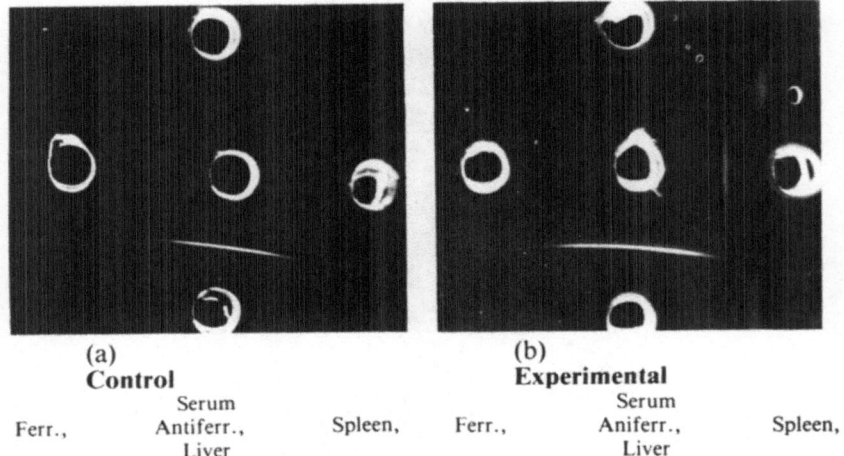

(a)
Control

Serum

Ferr.,   Antiferr.,   Spleen,

Liver

(b)
Experimental

Serum

Ferr.,   Aniferr.,   Spleen,

Liver

Figure 1 Agar immunodiffusion of adult rat tissue homogenates, the middle well contains the rat antiferritin serum. The native ferritin, tissue homogenate, and serum samples are placed on the periphery

the undiluted tissue homogenate against the antiferritin serum. It is interesting to note that the controls are negative, whereas the experimental samples are positive. The positive arc on the left is of native ferritin.

These preliminary immunological investigations prove interesting as the experimental macerates react against the antiferritin serum, showing that the molecule has undergone transport through the intestinal cells and has not been degraded or denatured, but has retained its antigenicity. Although the control samples show a slight positive reaction, probably due to a cross-reaction, the experimental samples are significantly higher. It is hoped to carry out further experiments both on the organs and also on lymph collected from the intestinal lymphatic, in these studies, it is hoped that enough lymph can be collected so that a concentrated solution can be obtained to carry out chromatographic studies, and also ultracentrifugation analysis. By these investigations we may find the proportion of native protein in the organs and the lymph.

Electronmicroscopic investigations

Ultrastructural examination following ferritin administration into the small intestine showed a pattern of absorption highly comparable to

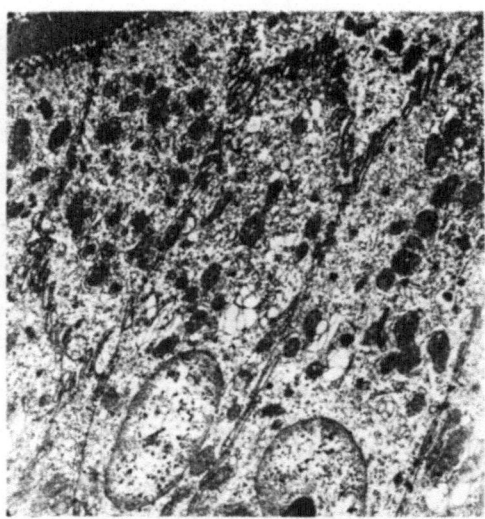

Figure 2 An electronmicrograph of a duodenal cell from a control adult rat. Many mitochondria are seen suggesting active and constant transport. Many fingerlike projections or microvilli are present, and this suggests a large absorption capacity for the cell. Osmium tetroxide fixation. × 3600

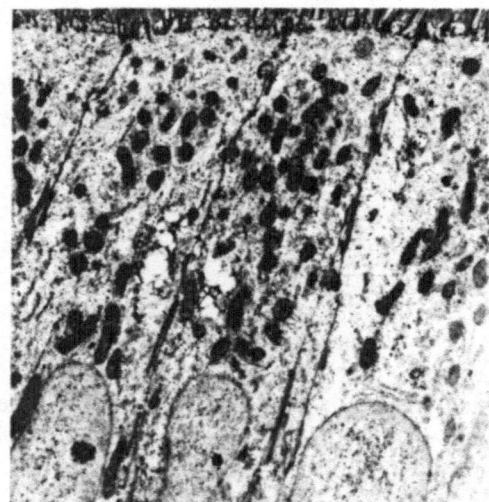

Figure 3 An electronmicrograph of a control ileal cell, the microvillous border is again present, mitochondria are seen in abundance. Note the similarity to the duodenal cells, and the difference between the neonatal ileum which contains many pinocytotic vacuoles. Osmium tetroxide fixation. × 3600

results of a previous study involving ligated segments of gut in the neonatal rat (Williams, 1974). In this present study the marker was seen to be adsorbed onto the apical surface membrane, and contained within cytoplasmic vesicular and vacuolar structures. Some free ferritin tracer was also observed. The gut mucosa withstood the experimental conditions very well and was very comparable to the normal adult rat intestine. To show the viability of the cell, low and high magnification micrographs are presented.

Figures 2 and 3 are micrographs of duodenal and ileal sections from the control animal, it can be seen that the tissue was not damaged in any way, fixation was good, except maybe for some slight swelling of a few mitochondria.

Figures 4-12 are experimental sections of duodenum and ileum from animals that had experienced ferritin injection. These micrographs depict the typical appearance of many micrographs studied, the presence of the tracer protein varied a little inasmuch as some cells contained more than others.

As with the quantitative data, the electronmicroscopic investigations demonstrate that there is passage of ferritin from the lumen into the intercellular spaces and lymphatics.

DISCUSSION

These studies using ferritin as a tracer marker indicate that a small, but significant amount of intraluminal protein traverses the mammalian gut, and reaches the intestinal lymph and other body organs intact.

In these experiments, ferritin was injected directly into ligated washed segments of duodenum and ileum, thereby avoiding any proteolytic activity of gastric enzymes; electronmicroscopic and immunological methods were employed. In the past the small intestine of the adult rat was thought to be impermeable to macromolecules, but with more modern methods, this has been found not to be so.

Detectable amounts of the tracer were transmitted from the lumen across the intestinal mucosa. Previous electronmicroscopic and immunological studies from this laboratory showed that passage of ferritin occurs from the lumen to the intercellular space and lymphatics of the neonatal rat (Williams, 1975). In these studies the tracer was taken up in membrane-bound vacuoles, and also by diffusion into the cell. In this study on the adult rat, employing virtually the same techniques, the tracer was observed in membrane-bound vacuoles, with

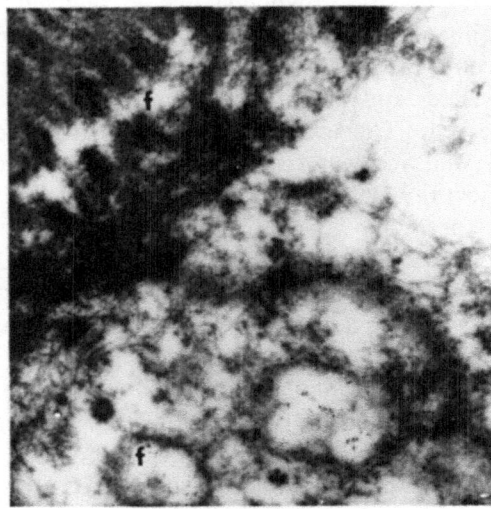

Figure 4 An electronmicrograph of a duodenal cell from an adult rat intestine after administration of ferritin. The protein can be seen in the lumen, and also taken up in vacuoles inside the cytoplasm. Osmium tetroxide fixation. × 24 000

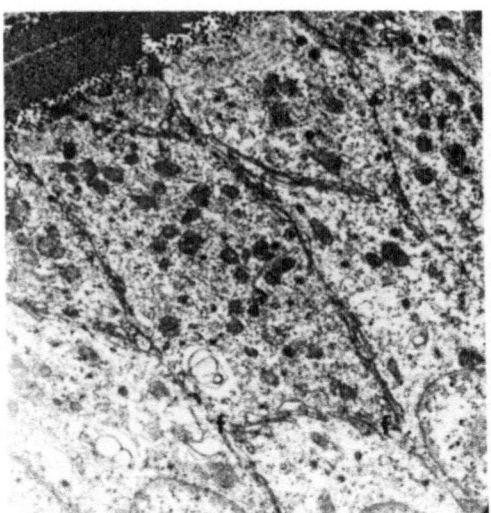

Figure 5 This is a low-power micrograph of Figure 6. Ferritin was identified in pockets in the intercellular spaces, showing that transport of this protein had occurred. Osmium tetroxide fixation. × 2400

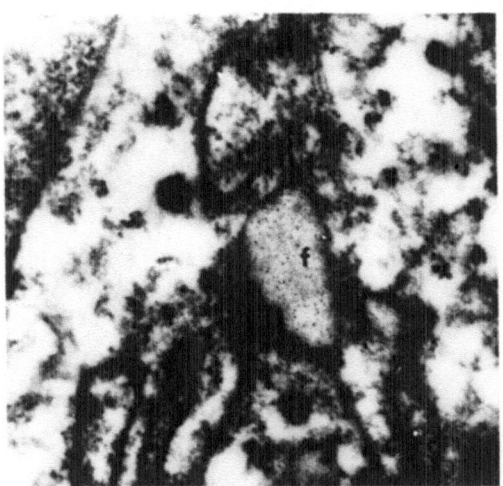

Figure 6 This is a micrograph of a magnified section of the intercellular space, showing the presence of ferritin. Some of the tracer was also observed free in the cytoplasm of the cell. Osmium tetroxide fixation. × 24 000

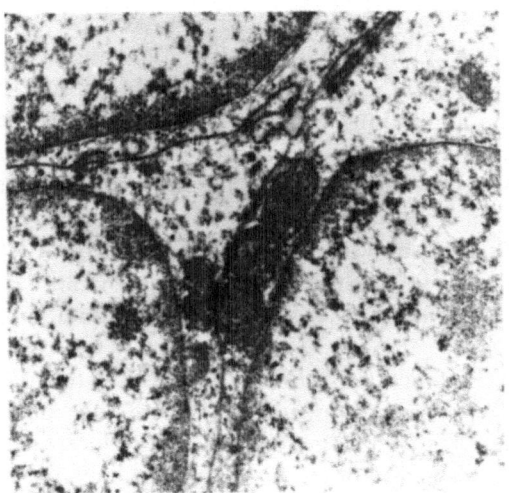

Figure 7 A low-power view of the intercellular space between two cells. Below the nuclei is the intercellular space containing the tracer, and at higher magnification, ferritin is seen in this space. Osmium tetroxide / gluteraldehyde fixation. × 3600

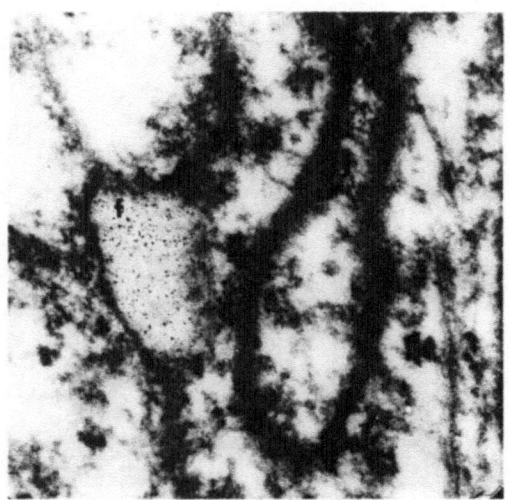

Figure 8 Is a magnified view of the previous micrograph. This shows a substantial amount of the tracer protein in the intercellular space. Osmium tetroxide / gluteraldehyde fixation. × 36 000

some free ferritin in the cytoplasm of the cell. In both cases, passage of ferritin into the intercellular space was observed. Other workers, namely, Warshaw et al., 1974; Kreahenbühl et al., 1969 and Walker et al., 1973 have observed also that there is macromolecular transport across the gut; using bovine serum albumin, ferritin, and horseradish peroxidase, these proteins were found in significant amounts. Horseradish peroxidase was shown to cross the adult mucosal cell in pinocytotic vesicles in a fashion identical with that observed with gamma-globulin in the neonatal stage. Bamford (1965) also showed that Salmonella antigen is taken into the adult rat. Bockman (1966) showed ferritin uptake and transport into the lamina propria of adult hamster after intraluminal administration of the protein.

Neonatal intestinal protein uptake and transport to the circulation has been shown to be of great importance in mammals that obtain passive immunity from colostrum (Brambell, 1970), but direct observation of macromolecular transport has been more difficult in the adult. Clark (1959) and others claimed that there was total cessation of transport of macromolecules soon after the closure or cut off period. This study disagrees with this and confirms the previously mentioned authors' investigations, that such passage can and does occur after cut-off. From

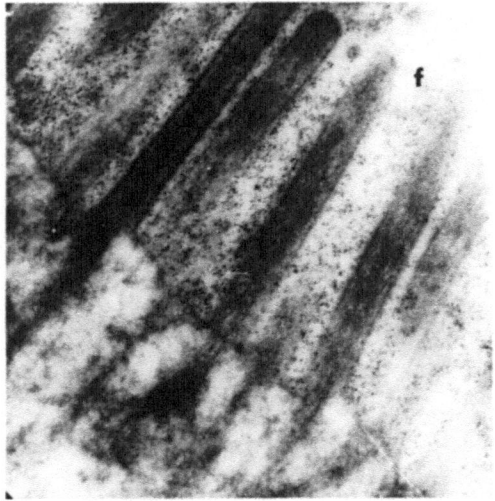

Figure 9 Electronmicrograph of an ileal section from a ferritin-fed animal. Ferritin is seen in abundance in the intestinal lumen, some is also seen inside the microvilli, and some is observed about to enter the cell at the base of the villi. Osmium tetroxide fixation. × 24 000

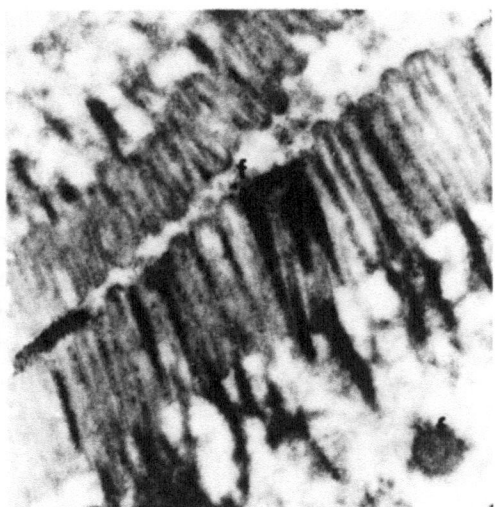

Figure 10 Ileal section of a ferritin fed adult rat. Ferritin can be seen in the lumen, and also in the region of the terminal web. The protein is contained mainly in membrane bound vacuoles. Osmium tetroxide fixation. × 15 000

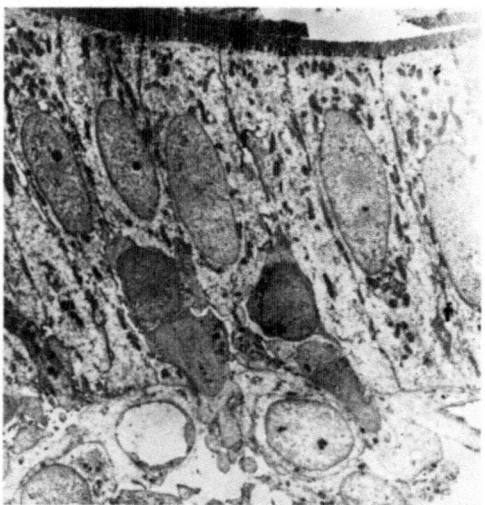

Figure 11 A low-power view of the ileal region of the ferritin-fed animal. The protein was observed in the intercellular space. Osmium tetroxide / gluteraldehyde fixation. × 1500

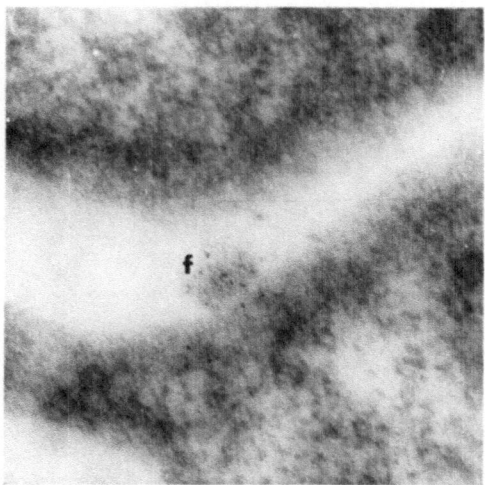

Figure 12 A high magnification of Figure 11. The tracer protein is clearly seen in the intercellular space, but not in great quantity. More was observed in the duodenal sections. Osmium tetroxide / gluteraldehyde fixation. × 36 000

the data obtained during the course of these preliminary investigations, it is shown that transmission of ferritin occurs across the rat mucosa. From the immunological data this seems to be a significant amount, and agrees with other studies (Hemmings, 1975 a, b). The uptake of ferritin by the duodenal cells is interesting, in so far that this proximal part of the intestine is thought to be more selective in the suckling (Rodewald, 1970; Jones, 1974; Hemmings and Williams, 1974) whereas the ileal, or distal region was thought to be more concerned in uptake and breakdown, (Hemmings and Williams, 1974; Hemmings, 1975).

Although the data are not quantitative, more intracellular ferritin was observed in the duodenal region in the present study. Ferritin was also observed in the cells in the ileal sections and intercellular spaces, so there was not a total breakdown of the protein. These results agree with previous observations on the neonate when cellular ferritin was observed in both the proximal and distal sections of the intestine (Williams, 1974).

The immunological tests did not show ferritin in the circulation, and this might be due to a dilution effect; however the values for the spleen and the liver were substantially higher than the values obtained for the control samples. These results also show that a proportion of the transmitted ferritin has retained its antigenicity. The intracellular proteolytic enzymes have not entirely degraded the protein during its passage through the cell.

Further knowledge of the mechanism involved in the transport of macromolecules from the lumen to the cell should be important in explaining the factors influencing absorption of these large molecules of pathophysiological significance, e.g. those that can stimulate immune response of allergic types following their ingestion. Ferritin is a useful tracer for macromolecular transport studies because it can be identified in more than one way.

These investigations have demonstrated that ferritin is a useful tracer for studies of the limited macromolecular absorption that occurs normally in the mature mammalian small intestine. There is variation in the immunological results, and some animals seem to transport more ferritin from the lumen than others. This is perhaps due to the body's requirement for iron varying from one animal to another.

The findings presented here confirm other workers observations of macromolecular transport in the adult intestine (Warshaw et al., 1974; Walker et al., 1973).

Further studies are planned to study the factors that might increase or suppress transmission of molecules across the small intestine of the adult.

References

Bamford, D. R. (1965). Studies in vitro of the passage of serum proteins across the gut wall of young rats. Thesis. (Univ. Wales.)

Brambell, F. W. R. (1970). The transmission of passive immunity from mother to young. (Amsterdam: North Holland).

Bockman, D. E. (1966). Light and electronmicroscopy of intestinal ferritin absorption. Observations in sensitized and nonsensitized hamsters. Anat. Rec., **155**, 603

Clark, S. L. (1959). The ingestion of proteins and colloidal material by columnar cells of the small intestine in suckling rats and mice. J. Biophys. Biochem. Cytol., **5**, 41

Cornell, R., Walker, W. A. and Isselbacher, K. J. (1971). Small intestinal absorption of horseradish peroxidase, a cytochemical study. Lab. Invest., **25**, 42

Hemmings, W. A. and Williams, E. W. (1974). Uptake of labelled ferritin and Rat IgG from segments of the gut of the suckling rat. I.R.C.S. Med.Sci., **2**, 1450

Hemmings, W. A. and Williams, E. W. (1975). Transport of ferritin across the ileum of suckling rats. I.R.C.S. Med.Sci., **3**, 215

Hemmings, W. A. (1975). Degradation products in gut and carcase tissue after injecting labelled ferritin into the ileum of suckling rats. I.R.C.S. Med.Sci., **3**, 216

Hemmings, W. A. (1975). Transport of protein across the small intestine of adult rats following injection of ferritin to the intestinal lumen. I.R.C.S. Med.Sci., **3**, 262

Jones, R. E. (1976). Studies on the transmission of bovine IgG across the intestine of the young rat. In: (W. A. Hemmings (ed.), Maternofoetal Transmission of Immunoglobulins, 323. (London: Cambridge University Press)

Kraehenbühl, J. P. and Campiche, M. A. (1969). Early stages of intestinal absorption of specific antibodies in the newborn; An ultrastructural, cytochemical, and immunological study in the pig, rat and rabbit. J. Cell. Biol., **42**, 343

Ouchterlony, O. (1958). Diffusion in gel, methods for immunological analysis. Prog. Allergy, **5**, 1

Palade, G. E. (1952). A study of fixation for electronmicroscopy. J. Exp. Med., **95**, 285

Pease, D. C. (1964). Histological Techniques for Electronmicroscopy. (New York: Academic Press)

Rodewald, R. (1970). Route of selective antibody transport in the small intestine of the neonatal rat. J. Cell. Biol., **43,** 118

Walker, W., Isselbacher, K. J. and Bloch, K. J. (1973). Intestinal uptake of macromolecules. J. Immunol., **111,** 221

Warshaw, A. L., Walker, A. and Isselbacher, K. J. (1974). Protein uptake by the intestine, evidence for absorption of intact molecules. Gastroenterology, **66,** 987

Williams, E. W. (1974). Uptake of ferritin in the gut of the suckling rat. I.R.C.S. Alim. System, **2,** 1341

Williams, E. W. (1974). An electronmicroscopic study of ferritin transport through the gut of the suckling rat. I.R.C.S. Alim. System, **2,** 1514

Williams, E. W. (1975). Protein transfer through rabbit foetal and neonatal rat membranes, Thesis. M. I. Biol.

7

Oral immunization of rats with human serum albumin: interference with intestinal absorption and tolerogenic effect

C. ANDRÉ, J. P. VAERMAN and J. F. HEREMANS

The first part of this communication deals with our previous data (André et al., 1974) concerning the inhibition of intestinal absorption of human serum albumin (HSA) in rats who had received a large dose of this antigen by intragastric intubation. The second part reports on the decreased immune response to parenteral administration of HSA displayed by rats orally immunized by the same procedure as that used in the first part.

INTERFERENCE OF ORAL IMMUNIZATION WITH INTESTINAL ABSORPTION

Conventional female Wistar rats weighing around 200 g were used throughout. Oral immunization was performed as follows: groups of five rats were fasted for 24 h, whereupon they were administered 200 mg of HSA in 2 ml of saline by gastric intubation. The test for intestinal absorption, performed 2 weeks after the priming dose, also consisted in a single intragastric administration of 200 mg of HSA after one day fasting. Mesenteric venous blood was obtained 1, 2 or 3 h later. Animals were devided into four groups, according to whether animals were or not primed, and were or not tested for absorption, as shown in Table 1. The concentration of HSA in the mesenteric venous serum, which reflects the

Table 1 Effects of oral immunization on intestinal absorption of HSA: subdivision of rats in four experimental groups

Experimental group	n	Oral immunization; 200 mg HSA intragastrically	Intestinal absorption test.: 200 mg HSA intragastrically	Meaning
I	5	—	—	Control or blank
II	15	—	+	Normal absorption
III	5	+	—	Residual HSA from oral immunization
IV	15	+	+	Inhibition of absorption

intestinal absorption, was measured both by an electrophoretic radio-immunoassay (RIA) and by single radial immunodiffusion.

The results, outlined in Table 2, clearly indicate that there was a significantly decreased absorption of HSA 2 weeks after a first oral dose of this antigen. The difference with control absorption was most pronounced at 1 h and 2 h after the test dose was given.

In order to confirm that this decreased absorption was the result of the presence, in the intestinal secretions of the orally primed animals, of substances capable of inhibiting the intestinal uptake of HSA, the following experiment of passive oral immunization was performed. Two groups of ten rats, who had never experienced any contact with HSA, were fasted for 24 h. Then, they received a test dose of 200 mg of iodine-125 labelled HSA (in one ml of 0.15 M bicarbonate containing 1600 units of pancreatic protease inhibitor). This test dose was mixed with scrapings of the small bowel mucosa of either unprimed or of intragastrically primed rats. The latter had received 200 mg of HSA by gastric intubation 2 weeks earlier. The absorption of the labelled HSA was assayed by measuring the non-dialysable radioactivity of venous mesenteric serum 2 hours after the test dose, mixed with the scrapings,

Table 2 Inhibition of intestinal absorption by active oral immunization

Group	Oral priming	Testing	Method of HSA titration	Concentration of HSA in mesenteric serum at various times after test dose (µg/ml)		
				1 h	2 h	3 h
I	—	—	RIA		0	
	—	—	SRI		0	
II	—	+	RIA	290	668	140
	—	+	SRI	102	443	84
III	+	—	RIA		140	
	+	—	SRI		0	
IV	+	+	RIA	10	40	38
	+	+	SRI	34	111	50

Table 3 Inhibition of intestinal absorption by passive oral immunization

Group	Intragastric intubation with scrapings of intestinal mucosa from	Test dose mixed with scrapings	Concentration of HSA in mesenteric serum 2 h after test dose ($\mu g/ml$)		
			Mean	SEM	Range
Control (n = 10)	Normal rats	0.2 mg HSA	41.8	2.6	31-53
Test (n = 10)	Rats orally immunized with HSA	0.2 mg HSA	27.2	1.8	21-32

was injected in the stomach. The results are presented in Table 3. The absorption of labelled HSA in the test groups was only 65% of that observed in the control group and this was a highly significant difference ($p<0.01$). Thus, it appears that the intestinal secretions and/or mucosa from rats who had received 200 mg of HSA by the intragastric route, contain substances capable of interfering with the absorption of HSA.

The next point was to verify whether these substances were antibodies and possibly IgA antibodies. Again, intestinal mucosa scrapings were obtained from rats orally immunized as above and from control rats. The scrapings were homogenized and centrifuged at high speed to remove insoluble matter consisting of cells, mucus and cellular fragments. The supernatant, containing the hypothetical secretory antibodies, was salted out with 50% saturated ammonium sulphate. The precipitate of intestinal globulins obtained after high speed centrifugation was redissolved in and dialysed against buffered saline. This solution was then passed over a column of Sepharose-bound HSA, prepared by the cyanogen bromide activation procedure of Cuatrecasas (1970). The intestinal globulins of control rats were similarly passed over an HSA Sepharose column of the same size. Both columns were then extensively washed with buffered saline, until the optical density of the effluent was near zero. Antibodies, if any, were then eluted with 3 M ammonium thiocyanate: after dialysis against buffered saline, they were concentrated to a volume of about 0.5 ml. When these concentrated samples were analysed by Ouchterlony tests using specific antisera against rat IgM or IgA (Vaerman et al., 1973), only the sample from the orally immunized rats gave rise to a precipitin line, and only with the anti-IgA antiserum. The amount of protein eluted from the HSA column for the control rats was very low, and whatever protein was present, it did not react with any of the anti-Ig antisera. These results support the presence of anti-HSA antibodies of IgA class in the intestinal mucosa and/or secretions of orally immunized rats.

Finally, immunohistological investigations were conducted on the intestinal mucosa of control and intragastrically immunized rats. Cryostat sections of jejunum were incubated first with a solution (10 mg/ml) of HSA in buffered saline. After several rinses with buffered saline, the sections were further incubated with fluorescein-labelled anti-HSA antibodies (Behringwerke A. G., Marburg). Control sections were only reacted with the fluorescent anti-HSA antiserum. Numerous anti-HSA containing immunocytes were detected in the sections of the mucosa of immunized rats. Control sections were devoid of fluorescein-labelled cells, as well as sections from mucosae of non-immunized control rats. The class of the Ig of these cells is now under investigation.

These data demonstrate that the administration of 200 mg of HSA in the stomach of adult rats results in the appearance of anti-HSA producing cells and IgA-antibodies in their intestinal mucosa, and that these antibodies interfere with the intestinal absorption of HSA.

TOLEROGENIC EFFECT OF ORAL IMMUNIZATION

Again, conventionel female Wistar rats were used (200 g). Animals were divided into three groups. Group A (n = 10) served as control and only received an intramuscular injection of 0.25 mg of HSA in Freund's incomplete adjuvant. Group B (n = 12) was first orally immunized by an intragastric administration of 200 mg of HSA in one ml of saline. Seven weeks later, the animals were challenged by the intramuscular route, as in group A. Group C (n = 10) was also first orally immunized, but the intramuscular challenge occurred only 23 weeks after the oral dose. The sera of all rats were collected 5 weeks after the intramuscular injection. Anti-HSA antibody in sera was assayed by their antigen-binding capacity (ABC 33), using iodine-125 labelled HSA and a 20% polyethylene glycol solution to separate free from antibody-bound HSA (Creighton et al., 1973). Results are expressed, in Table 4, as ug of bound HSA per ml of undiluted serum. There was a strong reduction in the anti-HSA antibody titres of group B rats, which had been orally primed 7 weeks before the parenteral challenge. Even group C rats had a significantly lower response than the control rats to a challenging parenteral immunization administered as late as 23 weeks after oral priming.

Table 4 Tolerogenic effect of oral immunization

Experimental group	Oral immunization 200 mg HSA intragastrically	Weeks before intramuscular challenge	Mean serum antigen binding capacity 5 weeks after challenge (μg HSA/ml)			p*
			Mean	SEM	Range	
A (n = 10)	—	—	260.0	6.5	231-285	< 0.001
B (n = 12)	+	7	60.0	21.8	2-191	< 0.001
C (n = 10)	+	23	225.5	8.1	191-258	< 0.005

*Significance (Student's t-test)

DISCUSSION

The first point which deserves discussion is the method of oral immunization, i.e. administration of a single large dose of antigen by intragastric intubation. It has been claimed that oral immunization of the rabbit to bovine serum albumin could be obtained in one day as well as in 30 days, provided the single dose was large enough (Rothberg et al., 1969). It remains to be established however whether one can generalize such a statement, and whether or not the levels of secretory antibodies would be comparable.

There was a large discrepancy between the levels of HSA in mesenteric serum measured by RIA and by SRI. This discrepancy was so high for the residual HSA 15 days after intragastric priming that doubts arose on the validity of the RIA used. It seems that the RIA of HSA was perturbed by material different from native HSA, but still reactive with anti-HSA antibodies. Such a material may consist in breakdown peptides of HSA, having retained some antigenic determinant(s) capable of binding to anti-HSA antibodies, but unable to precipitate with them.

The inhibition of intestinal absorption here reported may be more physiological than the in vitro studies on everted gut sacs (Walker et al., 1972; Walker et al., 1973; Levine et al., 1970). The fact that this inhibition was most marked during the first 2 hours of the test suggests that there was only enough intestinal antibody to deal with the first portions of the test dose of antigen.

The demonstration that intestinal scrapings of orally immunized animals contain only IgA antibodies, apparently produced by plasma cells of the gut mucosa, provides a logical explanation to the passive oral immunization here reported. The latter suggests that antigens in vitro precomplexed to secretory IgA antibodies are denied absorption by the gut wall. This supports the hypothesis that the major role of IgA antibodies in the gut is to prevent access of foreign antigenic material to the internal milieu.

Concerning the tolerogenic effect of oral immunization, it has long been known that oral administration of dinitrochlorobenzene or picrylchloride may prevent sensitization to the corresponding haptens (Chase, 1946), although no evidence was presented that digestive immunity was achieved.

Recently, a pronounced tolerogenic effect of oral immunization was reported for rats intubated with 25 mg of BSA daily for 14 days (Thomas and Parrott, 1974). However, in contrast with our studies, no antibodies nor antibody containing cells were found in the intestinal mucosa and secretions, although serum antibodies were present. The tolerogenic mechanism advanced was that of 'low zone' antigen induced tolerance, since it was demonstrated that minute amounts of native BSA got access to the circulation.

We are inclined to favour a mechanism relying on the tolerogenic effect of circulating IgA antibodies or of circulating Ag—IgA complexes. Preliminary evidence of the existence, in the sera of orally immunized rats, of antigen-antibody complexes has been obtained, using a sensitive test of inhibition of latex agglutination (Lurhuma et al., 1975), but these data require further confirmation. It is worth mentioning that antigen-antibody complexes have already been shown to be able to effect the blockade of effector antibody-producing cells (Schrader and Nossal, 1974).

ACKNOWLEDGEMENTS

This work was supported by Convention No. 74.7.0487 from the 'Délégation Générale à la Recherche Scientifique et Technique', Paris, and by grant No. 1192 from the Fonds de la Recherche Scientifique Médicale, Brussels, Belgium.

References

André, C., Lambert, R., Bazin, H. and Heremans, J. F. (1974). Interference of oral immunization with the intestinal absorption of heterologous albumin. Eur. J. Immunol., **4**, 701

Chase, M. W. (1946). Inhibition of experimental drug allergy by prior feeding of the sensitizing agent. Proc. Soc. Exp. Biol. Med., **61**, 257

Creighton, W. D., Lambert, P. H. and Meischer, P. A. (1973). Detection of antibodies and soluble antigen—antibody complexes by precipitation with polyethylene glycol. J. Immunol., **111**, 1219

Cuatrecasas, P. (1970). Protein purification by affinity chromatography. Derivitizations of agarose and polyacrylamide beads. J. Biol. Chem., **245**, 3059

Levine, R. R., McNary, W. F., Kornguth, P. J. and Le Blanc, R. (1970). Histological re-evaluation of everted gut technique for studying intestinal absorption. Eur. J. Pharmacol., **9**, 211

Lurhuma, A., Cambiaso, C. L., Masson, P. L. and Heremans, J. F. (1976). Detection of circulating antigen-antibody complexes by their inhibiting effect on the agglutination of IgG-coated particles by rheumatoid factor or Clq. I. Characterization of the inhibiting factors. Clin. Exp. Immunol., **25**, 212

Rothberg, R. M., Kraft, R. S., Farr, R. S., Kriebel, G. W. and Goldberg, S. S. (1969). Local immunologic responses to ingested protein, pp.293-307. In: (D. H. Dayton et al. (eds.) 'The Secretory Immunologic System', (Washington: U.S. Government Printing Office)

Schrader, J. W. and Nossal, G. J. V. (1974). Effector cell blockade. A new mechanism of immune hyporeactivity induced by multivalent antigens. J. Exp. Med., **139**, 1582

Thomas, H. C. and Parrott, D. M. (1974). The induction of tolerance to a soluble protein antigen by oral administration. Immunology, **27**, 631

Vaerman, J. P., André, C., Bazin, H. and Heremans, J. F. (1973). Mesenteric lymph as a major source of serum IgA in guinea-pigs and rats. Eur. J. Immunol., **3**, 580

Walker, W. A., Isselbacher, K. J. and Bloch, K. J. (1972). Intestinal uptake of macromolecules. I Effect of oral immunization. Science, **177**, 608

Walker, W. A., Isselbacher, K. J. and Bloch, K. J. (1973). Intestinal uptake of macromolecules. II Effect of parenteral immunization. J. Immunol., **111**, 221

8

Biological function of antigen—IgA antibody complexes: in vivo and in vitro interference with intestinal absorption and tolerogenic effect

C. ANDRÉ, F. ANDRÉ and J. P. VAERMAN

We previously reported that rats, immunized orally (intragastrically) with 200 mg human serum albumin (HSA) displayed a significantly decreased serum antibody response to a subsequent parenteral injection of HSA (André et al., 1977). In addition, such rats had a reduced intestinal absorption of a tracer dose of HSA (André et al., 1974). Anti-HSA antibodies of the IgA class were detected in their intestinal secretions as well as in the cytoplasm of some of their gut plasma cells, as shown by immunofluorescence (André et al., 1977). Moreover, when a test dose of labelled HSA was mixed with intestinal secretions from orally immunized rats, there was a significant decrease of the absorption of the labelled HSA as compared to that of the same dose mixed with normal intestinal contents (André et al., 1974).

The present data deal with the inhibitory effect of a mouse anti-DNP IgA-antibody on the intestinal absorption of DNA-HSA.

Furthermore, we have attempted the characterization of a factor present in the serum of mice intragastrically immunized 2 weeks earlier with sheep red blood cells (SRBC). This factor was able to 'paralyse' specifically the secretion of direct anti-SRBC plaque forming cells taken from spleens of mice immunized intraperitoneally with SRBC 4 days earlier (André et al., 1975).

In vivo inhibition of intestinal absorption of iodine-125 labelled DNP-HSA by mouse MOPC-315 IgA

The MOPC-315 IgA myeloma protein was used as anti-DNP antibody (Eisen et al., 1968). Each mouse of three groups of ten (BALB/c) received 1 mg of iodine-125 labelled DNP-HSA antigen in 0.5 ml of 0.1 M sodium bicarbonate by the intragastric route. Two groups received the antigen mixed either with 1 mg of MOPC-315 IgA, an amount estimated to be close to equivalence, or with 0.25 mg IgA. Another group of ten mice received 1 mg of MOPC-315 IgA in 0.5 ml bicarbonate containing 1 mg of labelled HSA, devoid of DNP hapten. The purified MOPC-315 mouse IgA was supplied by Bionetics, Kensington, Md. Two hours after intragastric administration of the labelled antigen, the mice were exsanguinated and the TCA-precipitable radioactivity of their serum was measured. The amount of absorbed antigen was expressed as μg of TCA-precipitable radioactivity per ml of serum. The results (Table 1) show that only 1 mg of MOPC-315 IgA did significantly interfere with the intestinal absorption of DNP-HSA.

In vitro inhibition of intestinal absorption of iodine-125 labelled DNP-HSA by MOPC-315 IgA

Two everted gut sacs (5 cm of washed jejunum) were prepared from each of seven BALB/c mice. They were placed in 5 ml of Ringer's solution which had been previously admixed with 0.5 mg of iodine-125 labelled DNP-HSA with or without 0.125 mg of anti-DNP MOPC-315 IgA. After incubation for 1 h at 37 °C, the sacs were briefly rinsed in two successive baths of saline, opened, and their contents flushed with 2 ml

Table 1 In vivo inhibition of intestinal absorption of iodine-125 labelled DNP-HSA by anti-DNP MOPC-315 IgA myeloma protein

Number of mice (BALB/c)	Iodine-125 labelled protein in 0.5 ml of 0.1 M bicarbonate	MOPC-315 IgA mixed with labelled protein	Absorbed antigen: μg TCA-precipitable radioactivity per ml of serum
10	1 mg DNP-HSA	—	1.50* ± 0.27
10	1 mg DNP-HSA	0.25 mg IgA	1.69 ± 0.26
10	1 mg DNP-HSA	1 mg IgA**	0.45 ± 0.05
10	1 mg HSA	1 mg IgA	1.73 ± 0.25

*mean ± SD
**this amount of IgA is roughly equivalent to 1 mg DNP-HSA

74

Table 2 In vitro inhibition of intestinal (everted gut sacs) absorption of iodine-labelled DNP-HSA by MOPC-315 IgA

Number of mice	Labelled antigen in 5 ml Ringer	MOPC-315 IgA mixed with the labelled antigen	Absorbed antigen: nanograms of radioactive antigen per mg dry weight per hour
7	500 μg	—	8.3* $\pm$ 1.6
7	500 μg	125 μg	4.6 $\pm$ 1.3

* mean $\pm$ SD

of saline before being precipitated with TCA. The rinsed sacs were dried in the oven at 105 °C and weighed. The amount of antigen absorbed was estimated by counting the TCA-precipitate and it was expressed as nanograms of labelled antigen per mg of sac dry weight per hour (Table 2).

Again, the MOPC-315 IgA significantly decreased the intestinal absorption of DNP-HSA.

Immunochemical nature of the 'paralysing' factor

Spleen cells were collected from BALB/c mice which had been intra-peritoneally injected 4 days earlier with 2×10^8 SRBC. Before being plated for direct PFC, the spleen cells (25×10^6 in 0.5 ml) were incubated for 30 min at 37 °C with 0.5 ml of the following mixtures: (1) tissue culture medium; (2) normal mouse serum; (3) 'paralysing' serum, i.e. serum collected 15 days after 4 daily intragastric doses of 4×10^9 SRBC; (4) 'paralysing' serum which had been passed through a small column of Sepharose-bound rabbit rheumatoid factor (3); (5) 'paralysing' serum passed through a column of insolubilized goat anti-mouse- α- chain or (6) anti-mouse-μ-chain IgG antibodies; and (7) 'paralysing' serum absorbed on a column of insolubilized rabbit anti-SRBC IgG. For (5), (6) and (7), about 5 ml of immunoabsorbant (16 mg IgG per ml gel) were used per ml of serum. After passing through the various immunoabsorbents; the serum was reconcentrated to its original volume.

After incubation of the spleen cells in the various media, they were centrifuged 5 min at 200 g at room temperature and resuspended in 0.5 ml culture medium before being plated for direct PFC as previous described (André et al., 1975).

Results are listed in Table 3. Incubation with native 'paralysing' serum

Table 3 Characterization of 'paralysing' factor present in serum from mice intragastrically immunized with SRBC

Spleen cells, on day 4 after intraperitoneal injection of 2 × 10⁸ SRBC, incubated for 30 min at 37 °C with the following media, prior to plating for direct PFC	Number of spleen cell suspensions tested	Direct anti-SRBC PFC per 10⁶ spleen cells
(1) Eagle's tissue culture medium + 20% fetal calf serum	8	150* ± 10
(2) Normal mouse serum	7	190 ± 10
(3) 'paralysing' serum**	8	30 ± 7
(4) Same as (3), but absorbed on insolubilized rheumatoid factor to remove immune complexes	7	147 ± 23
(5) Same as (3), but after removal of IgA by insolubilized anti-mouse-α-chain antibodies	8	138 ± 14
(6) Same as (3), but after removal of IgM by insolubilized anti-mouse-μ-chain antibodies	8	31 ± 4
(7) Same as (3), but after passage through a column of insolubilized anti-SRBC antibodies	4	151 ± 20

*mean ± SD
**serum of mice taken 15 days after 4 daily intragastric administrations of 4 × 10⁹ SRBC

or with the same serum passed through the anti-μ-chain column profoundly 'paralysed' the secretion of IgM anti-SRBC by the spleen cells, as shown by a drastic decrease in the number of direct PFC when compared to incubation with culture medium or normal mouse serum. However, when the 'paralysing' serum had been passed through insolubilized rheumatoid factor, or insolubilized anti-mouse-α-chain- or anti-SRBC- antibodies, its 'paralysing' activity was removed, as shown by the large numbers of PFC obtained.

Molecular size of the 'paralysing factor'

Gel-filtration of 5 ml of 'paralysing' serum was performed on a 100 × 2.5 cm column of Ultrogel AcA 22 (LKB). The elution profile and the agarose gel electrophoresis of the six pooled concentrated (to 3.5 ml) fractions are illustrated in Figure 1. Each fraction was then dialysed against culture medium and assessed for its 'paralysing' activity, as

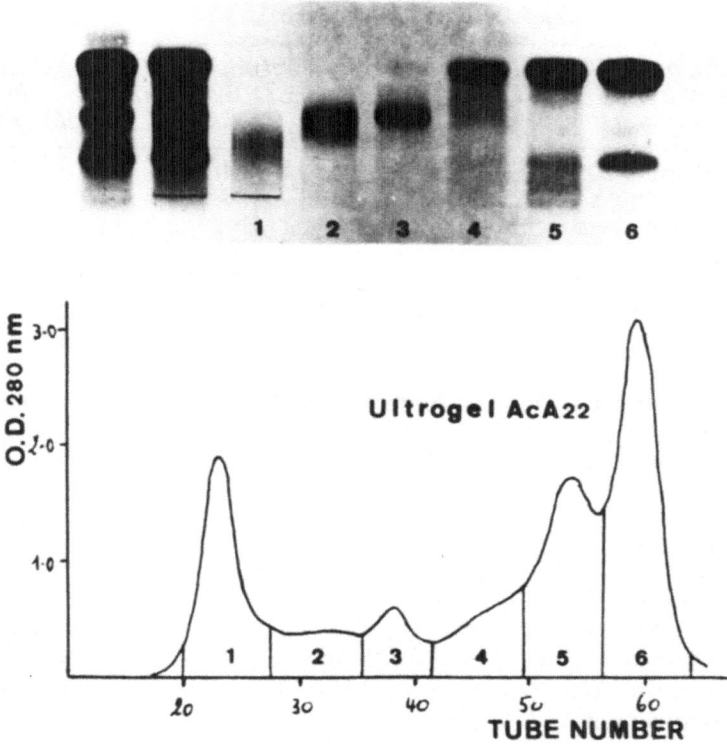

Figure 1 Gel-filtration of 5 ml of 'paralysing' serum on Ultrogel AcA22. Bottom: elution profile. Top: agarose gel electrophoresis of normal serum (extreme left), 'paralysing' serum and successive Ultrogel fractions 1 to 6, from left to right. Anode to the top.

compared to the original serum and culture medium by incubation with spleen cells taken from a mouse immunized intraperitoneally 4 days earlier with 2×10 SRBC. Results are shown in Table 4, as well as our estimation of the relative Ig content of each fraction, obtained by Ouchterlony analysis using specific antisera against mouse μ-, α- and β-chains. It is apparent that no single fraction displayed an activity comparable to that of the original serum. However, some 'paralysing' activity was clearly associated with fractions 3 to 6, with a maximum at fraction 5. This apparently correlated better with the IgG content of the fractions than with their IgA content.

77

Table 4 Molecular size of 'paralysing' factor, estimated from gel-filtration on ultrogel AcA22 (see Figure 1)

Spleen cells, on day 4 after intraperitoneal injection of 2 × 10^8 SRBC, incubated with the following media prior to plating	Direct anti-SRBC PFC/10^6 spleen cells	Relative content* in		
		IgM	IgA	IgG
Eagle's medium + 20% fetal calf serum	184**			
Original 'paralysing' serum	48			
Ultrogel Fraction 1(see Figure 1)	161	+	+	−
2	169	+ +	+	−
3	135	−	+ +	+
4	102	−	+ +	+ +
5	83	−	+	+ + +
6	131	−	−	+

*estimated by semiquantitative Ouchterlony analysis using monospecific antisera
**mean of 4 cell suspensions tested

DISCUSSION

Our first data demonstrate some function of IgA antibodies in specific inhibition of the intestinal absorption of antigens. They are consonant with our previous results obtained with intestinal secretions of rats orally immunized with HSA (André et al., 1974). They are also in agreement with recent data of Stokes, Soothill and Turner (1975), who studied the inhibition of absorption of DNP-HSA through the rat respiratory tract by the anti-DNP MOPC-315 IgA protein. However, it might seem desirable in such studies to use more 'physiological' IgA-antibodies, i.e. secretory IgA antibodies (IgA containing the secretory component). These have been shown to be more resistant to the adverse conditions prevailing in the exocrine secretions. The recent characterization of the SC of the mouse by our group (unpublished results) may be a significant progress in this direction.

The second part of this report deals with a preliminary characterization of the factor, present in the serum of mice orally (intragastrically) immunized with SRBC, which is able to 'paralyse' the expression of direct IgM PFC. In a previous study (André et al., 1975), we reported that such a serum inhibited slightly (to a titre of 1/8) the agglutination of human IgG-coated latex particles by rabbit rheumatoid factor. Since low titres of IgA anti-SRBC existed in such sera, it was hypothesized that the 'paralysing' factor might be a soluble immune complex with IgA antibodies involved. The removal of the 'paralysing' factor from the serum by columns of insolubilized rabbit rheumatoid factor, anti-mouse-α-chain antibodies or anti-SRBC IgG, but not by insolubilized anti-mouse-μ-chain antibodies are in support of this hypothesis.

However, the gel-filtration experiment does not seem to be compatible with it, since there was no correlation of 'paralysing' activity with the presence of large molecular size IgA. One cannot exclude, nevertheless, that monomeric IgA molecules might be involved having their combining sites occupied by small antigenic determinants of the SRBC membrane. However, such complexes appear completely different from those described by Schrader and Nossal (1974). The latter authors reported that immune complexes (IgG antibody) in slight antigen excess were powerful 'paralysers' of direct PFC, by representing a highly multivalent form of antigen and blocking the antibody secretion of the PFC ('Effector cell blockade').

Further investigations on the nature, appearance and persistance of this 'paralysing' factor in the serum of orally immunized mice are now in progress.

ACKNOWLEDGEMENTS

This work was supported by grants No. 74.7.0487 from the Délégation Générale à la Recherche Scientifique et Technique, Paris: No. 1192 from the Fonds de la Recherche Scientifique Médicale, Brussels. Financial assistance from the Fonds Cancérologique de la Caisse Générale d'Epargne et de Retraite, Brussels, is also acknowledged.

References

André, C., Heremans, J. F. Vaerman, J. P. and Cambiaso, C. L. (1975). A mechanism for the induction of immunological tolerance by antigen feeding: Antigen-antibody complexes. J. Exp. Med., **142**, 1509

André, C., Lambert, R., Bazin, H. and Heremans, J. F. (1974). interference of oral immunisation with intestinal absorption of heterologous albumin. Eur. J. Immunol., **4**, 701

André, C., Vaerman, J. P. and Heremans, J. F. (1977). This volume p.67

Eisen, H. N., Simms, E. S. and Potter, M. (1968). Mouse myeloma proteins with anti-hapten activity. The protein produced by plasma cell tumor MOPC-315. Biochemistry, **7**, 4126

Schrader, J. W. and Nossal G. J. V. (1974). Effector cell blockade. A new mechanism of immune hyporeactivity induced by multivalent antigens. J. Exp. Med., **139,** 1582

Stokes, C. R., Soothill, J. F. and Turner, M. W. (1975). Immune exclusion is a function of IgA. Nature, 255, 745

9

Antibody response in pigs and calves to antigens from the intestinal lumen and the efficacy of oral immunoprophylaxis against post-weaning enteric infection

P. PORTER and W. D. ALLEN

Modern agriculture has become increasingly reliant on the use of antibiotics routinely to maintain good animal performance in intensive rearing systems. The subsequent decline in efficiency and occurrence of disease associated with drug resistance (Smith, 1960) caused a re-evaluation of their use, and the eventual adoption of the recommendations of the Swann Committee Report (1969) was viewed with considerable alarm being estimated to have a potential cost to British Agriculture of approximately £30 million per annum. The prospect of equating antibodies rather than antibiotics with animal health is a serious goal for all conservationists and the now universal concern to restrict the use of antibiotics for the more serious health problems makes immunoprophylaxis of animal diseases an urgent objective.

Enteric disorders in the young animal represent a major proportion of farm disease problems. These commonly occur during periods of stress associated with changes in the animal's pattern of behaviour. At weaning, in particular, most animals are susceptible to a diarrhoea which is frequently exacerbated by a rapid proliferation of E.coli. For example, it is quite normal practice for a young calf to be removed from its dam as early as 4 days of age and be transported to a different farm for rearing on an artificial milk substitute. The stress of transport, change of environment, as well as weaning from maternal milk present a severe challenge to a young animal which has had very little experience of an extra-uterine environment. Indeed, Smith (1962) has suggested that in any consideration of diarrhoea syndromes, the question that may be rightly asked is not why do calves so reared become ill, but rather how do most of them survive.

Although the predisposing factors in the pathogenesis of post-weaning enteric syndromes are complex, one factor — the withdrawal of the protective function of maternal milk — is of signal importance. This, together with the stress resulting from the removal of the animal from the maternal environment is usually sufficient to promote a dramatic change in the intestinal microflora. The period of approximately 2 weeks following weaning is a critical one, during which the animal may show an alarming deterioration in health.

ANTIBODY FORMATION AND DEVELOPMENT DURING THE NEONATAL PERIOD

In young pigs and calves, the alimentary tract is probably the first organ to encounter major antigenic challenge, through the ingestion of micro-organisms whilst suckling. The impact of colonization of the gastrointestinal tract by bacteria is reflected by the profound changes which occur in its morphology during the early life of the animal. Survival and subsequent health of these animals may be largely determined by a successful inter-relationship between an early onset of active immunoglobulin synthesis, compensating for the steady decline in maternally derived passive antibody.

In both species passively derived circulating anti-E.coli antibodies have fallen to an ineffectual level by the time the animal is 10-days-old, but actively synthesized serum antibody does not reach an effective level until they are some 4-5 weeks of age. Thus, there is a period during which the animal is heavily dependent on maternal antibody in the lumen.

A local intestinal secretory immune system mediated by an immunoglobulin analogous to human IgA has been defined in both the pig (Porter and Allen, 1969; Vaerman, 1970; Atkins, Schofield and Reeders, 1971) and the bovine (Porter and Noakes, 1970; Butler, Kiddy, Maxwell, Hylton and Asofsky, 1971). In both species the secreted immunoglobulin has all the physico-chemical properties of human 11S

IgA with free as well as bound secretory component being detected in the secretions. However, although considerable emphasis has been placed on IgA, because of its relative abundance in intestinal secretions, other immunoglobulins have been comparatively neglected. Moreover most studies have been conducted on animals which can be regarded as being immunologically mature.

In the newborn animal, there are very few lymphoid cells in the intestinal lamina, and lymphoid follicles are poorly defined. Consequent upon the development of a gut microflora the lamina becomes infiltrated with lymphocytes and plasma cells. Many of these are involved in producing IgM and during the first few weeks of life IgM cells are often numerically predominant over IgA. (Allen and Porter, 1973). We regard the contribution of IgM acting in concert with IgA as being particularly important at this time.

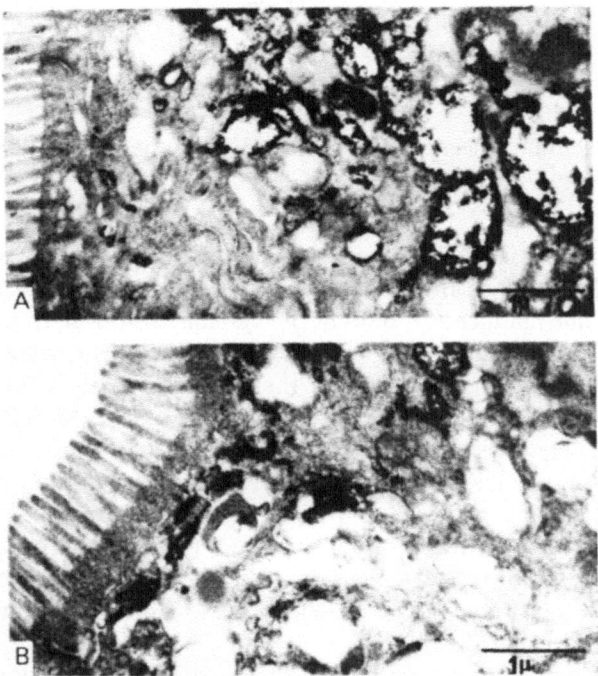

Figure 1 Electron micrographs of pig intestinal tissue treated with peroxidase conjugated rabbit anti-α-chain (A) anti-μ-chain (B) and hydrogen peroxide 3,3,diaminobenzidine followed by osmium tetroxide fixation. Each immunoglobulin is localized in numerous vesicles in the epithelial cell cytoplasm

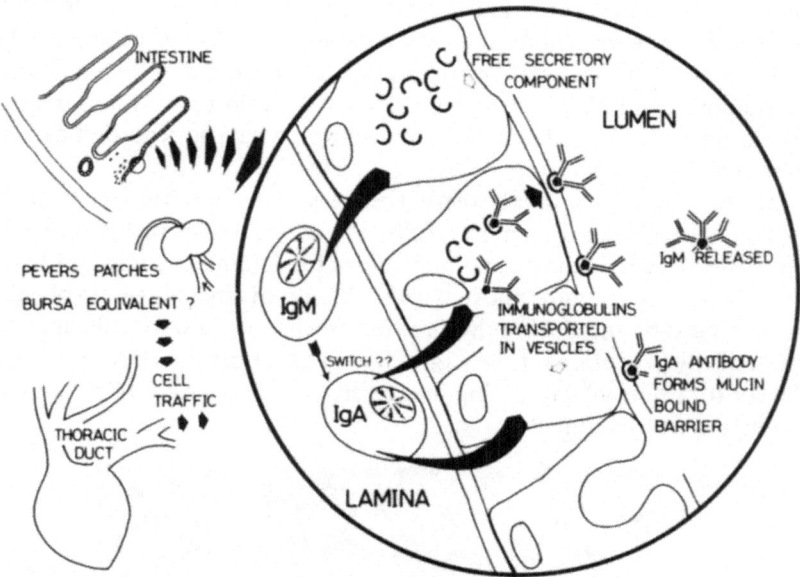

Figure 2 Cellular mechanisms involved in sythesis and transport of immunoglobulin in the intestinal mucosa

Furthermore it is possible that IgM plays an initiating role in the onset of antibody response in the mammalian exocrine immune system, in much the same manner as it does in the systemic response to parenterally administered antigens (Allen and Porter, 1973). The observation of Cebra (1969) gives support to this thesis in that rabbits infected with Trichinella showed a relative increase in intestinal IgM cells during a period 7-13 days post infection. Also in germ free mice, the repeated injection of anti-μ-chain antiserum causes a decrease in numbers of IgM cells in the lamina propria of the gut; a finding consistent with IgM producing cells being the precursors of IgA (Lawson, Asofsky, Hylton and Cooper, 1972). It is also significant that the exocrine role of IgA is taken over by IgM in cases of IgA deficiency (Stobo and Tomasi, 1967; Eidelman and Davies, 1968).

Immunoelectron microscopical studies on the localization of both immunoglobulins in crypt epithelial tissue suggest that the mechanism of transport for both is essentially similar. Many vesicles, containing either IgM or IgA were found in the apical cytoplasm of epithelial cells (Figure 1) and it is suggested that the immunoglobulin is transported across the epithelium by a process of reverse pinocytosis (Allen, Smith and Porter, 1973). In recent studies of human tissues (Poger and Lamm, 1974; Brandtzaeg, 1974) histological localization of free and bound secretory component favour a model in which 11S IgA is assembled in the epithelial cell.

Perhaps the function ascribed to secretory component, which is of particular interest in the present context however, is its affinity for mucin. This ensures that secreted antibody is bound in high local concentration to the surface of the villous epithelium, thus erecting an effective local barrier to infection. It is particularly interesting to note that the intestinal secretions of the preruminant calf contain higher levels of IgM than IgA mainly because the IgM is less effectively bound to the mucin and therefore more readily released into the lumen. (Porter, Noakes and Allen, 1972).

The reported observations relating to synthesis and secretion of immunoglobulins are shown in a schematic representation (Figure 2) with the purpose of conveniently summarizing known mechanisms concerned with the maintenance of integrity and function of the intestinal mucosa.

LOCAL ANTIBODY RESPONSE IN THE INTESTINE

The poor performance of parenteral vaccines in controlling enteritis has been widely noted. It appeared to us that the best prospect for initiating an adequate defence in the host to cope with the bacterial infections associated with weaning lay in exploiting the intestinal secretory immune mechanism by oral immunization.

Other studies of oral immunization have used faecal antibodies as an index of local intestinal response, but this provides no information about the antibody activity in any specific region of the alimentary tract. We have used animals, surgically prepared with Thiry-Vella loops, to study in detail, the secretory antibody response to bacterial antigens locally applied to the intestinal mucosa. The loop provides access to intestinal secretions without contamination from other sources such as saliva, bile, or gastric secretions. Intestinal secretion may be collected daily by attaching a polythene bag to the lower canula, or by irrigation with saline and collecting the washings. Biopsy speciments may be conveniently obtained using a peroral biopsy capsule, introduced into the canula, facilitating the immunohistological evaluation of the sequential changes at a cellular level. The loop retains all the normal intestinal function, having an intact blood and nerve supply. It retains its absorbtive and

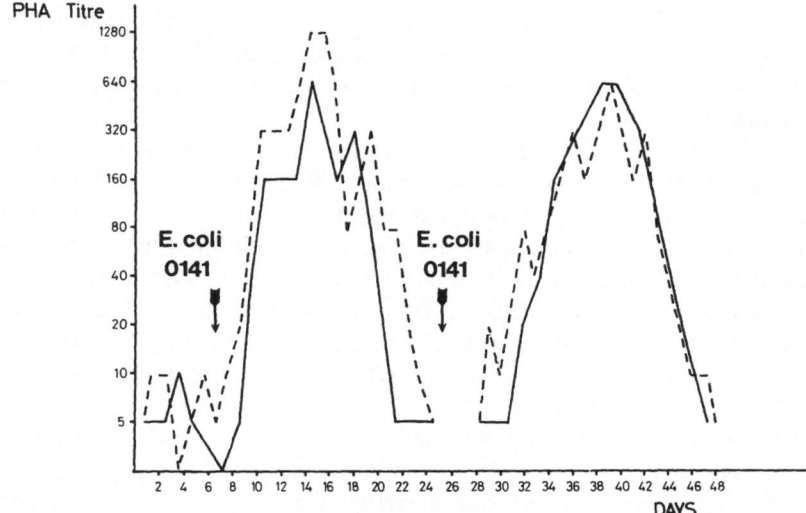

Figure 3 Secretion of antibodies in pig and calf in response to local application of heat inactivated E.coli 0141 antigen in Thiry-Vella loops. Pig—, Calf---

secretory function as well as peristaltic propulsion. It is therefore ideal in many respects for the study of secretory antibody responses to antigens applied locally to the intestinal mucosa.

Studies in both fistulated baby pigs and calves have shown that the appearance of antibodies in intestinal secretions can be stimulated by local application of heat inactivated E.coli antigens within the first 3 weeks of life, thus providing the basis for enhancing the competence of the young animal to cope with the challenge of enteropathogens after weaning (Porter, Kenworthy, Noakes and Allen, 1974; Allen and Porter, 1975). It is interesting to note that in the secretions from the fistulated calves, the levels of IgM frequently exceeded those of IgA demonstrating the important role of this immunoglobulin in the early stages of local intestinal immunity. Immunofluorescent studies of intestinal tissues from young pre-ruminant calves showed the presence of two main populations of immunocytes synthesizing IgM and IgA. These cells infiltrated the mucosa as early as 4 days of age and oral administration of antigen to colostral-fed calves of this age produced a copro-antibody response showing that active intestinal secretion could be successfully stimulated to inter-relate with a declining passive

86

antibody level (Allen and Porter, 1975).

In neither species however, did the intestinal antibody secretion persist for more than 3-4 weeks. A second dose of the same antigen induced an almost identical short lived response, similar in both intensity and duration (Figure 3). The characterization of the intestinal secretory antibody response were remarkably similar in pig and calf. In order to maintain consistent antibody secretion it was necessary to apply repeated doses. This apparent lack of memory in the secretory immune system, in contrast to that normally associated with systemic immunity has also been reported by other workers. (Ogra and Karzon, 1969). Freter and Gangarosa (1963) have previously recorded essentially similar observations in relation to oral immunization with heat-killed V. cholerae in which repeated doses were necessary for the maintenance of detectable levels of coproantibody. In this respect it is significant that Mattioli and Tomasi (1973) have recorded that intestinal IgA plasma cells in mice have a half life of only 4.7 days indicating that they do not play a significant role in long term memory, and suggesting that the persistence of antibody production would depend on the recruitment of further immunocompetent cells.

The requirement for the antigen to be administered in repeated doses can best be met, in the farm situation, by dietary inclusion. This ensures that the animal receives a dose of antigen with every feed, and additionally saves the labour of individual dosing. There was a practical problem in applying this concept to piglets, their intake of feed before weaning can be very variable. However it proved possible to add the heat-inactivated E.coli antigens to the diets at levels which ensure that on average, piglets consumed at least 10-30 times the minimum daily dose required (Porter, Kenworthy, Holme and Horsefield, 1973). With calves, which are given regulated feeds of milk replacer, this problem did not arise.

EVALUATION OF ORAL IMMUNIZATION AGAINST ENTERIC INFECTION AND ITS EFFECT ON GROWTH PERFORMANCE

Clinical studies were carried out in young pigs, experimentally infected with a virulent enteropathogenic E.coli 0149. Intestinal colonization of the orally immunized animals was delayed, and clinical symptoms were reduced both in intensity and duration, and generally there was a more rapid clearance of the infecting organisms than in the control animals.

Improved health was also reflected in terms of fewer deaths, better weight gains and food conversion ratios during the critical 2 week period post weaning. Parenteral immunization experiments provided no comparable benefits (Porter, Kenworthy and Allen, 1974).

In pilot trials with pigs housed in a conventional farm environment, the antigen fed animals also showed a reduction in the natural excretion of pathogenic E.coli compared with controls. Significant weight advantages were also recorded in the test pigs during the post weaning period. Furthermore, this was most effective in the smaller pigs. In litters with individual weights distributed below average at weaning, the antigen fed animals showed a significantly greater gain of 1.4 lb (0.6 kg) per pig (p < 0.01) in the first 2 weeks after weaning (Porter et al., 1973).

Extensive field trials on conventional farms affirmed the value of the concept in its wider application. The parameters selected to assess the efficacy of the treatment in this situation were those which would be most meaningful to the farmer, and consequently, more readily recognised and faithfully recorded. They included weight gain, food consumption, scouring pattern and medication. Significant benefits in

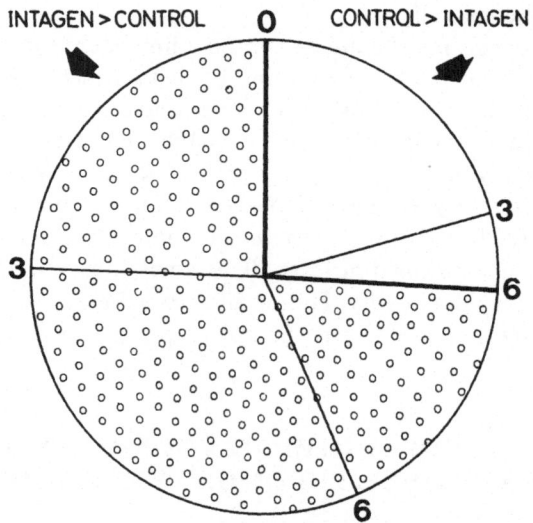

Proportion of litters showing weight advantages within limits
0 to 3, 3 to 6, and greater than 6 lbs per pig.

165 LITTERS

Figure 4 Proportional distribution of litters by weight comparing orally immunized pigs with controls

weight gain were a consistent feature of animals on the oral immunization regimen. The proportional advantages in trials with more than 3000 pigs are shown in Figure 4; the average weight advantage was 2.22 lb (0.99 kg) per pig (p<0.01) at 8 weeks of age.

The calf trials were conducted somewhat differently from those of the pig. Roy and his colleagues (1955) observed a significant deterioration in health and performance in successive batches of calves reared in units under continuous occupation. This was a consistent feature in the rearing of weaned calves over a period of 5 years and was a problem associated with certain pathogenic strains of E.coli.

We adopted this model system to evaluate the beneficial effects of oral immunization in calves (Porter, Kenworthy and Thompson, 1975). Strains of E.coli and Salmonella most commonly encountered in enteric disorders of calves were used to prepare the vaccine, which was included in the liquid milk substitute diets. The animals were housed in two identical units, and occupation of the units was continuous. This was achieved by staggering the intakes of calves, which were purchased in batches of 12. They were blocked in pairs according to weight and divided between the two rooms so that each incoming batch, some 2 weeks later, filled the remaining accommodation and subsequent batches immediately occupied the positions vacated by previous animals. The length of occupancy of each intake was 5 weeks; the trial lasted 12 months and 16 batches of animals passed through the units.

Animals in one unit were fed on the control diet and the others were fed on the same diet incorporating heat inactivated bacterial antigens.

Table 1 Oral immunization of the calf with bacterial antigens : effect on health and performance

Treatment	No. calves	Incidence scouring		Incidence treatment		Weight gain kg 0—5 weeks
		No. calves	No. days	Medicament	Antibiotic	
Control	96	50	142	52	31	13.04
Antigen	96	27*	50*	25*	11*	14.48**

* p<0.0
** p<0.0

For each batch of animals throughout the trials it was almost a consistent feature that the incidence of diarrhoea in the orally immunized group was considerably lower than in the controls, its duration was reduced and the requirements for treatment with either antibiotics or other medicaments were significantly reduced (Table 1). In consequence there were significant improvements in appetite and weight gain. It is interesting to note that most of the health problems occurred during the first 3 weeks of a calf's occupancy, a finding consistent with that of Roy et al. (1955) but most importantly the overall deterioration in performance shown in the control groups was practically abolished by oral immunization.

CONCLUSION

To conclude, progress in the development and use of oral enteric bacterial vaccines was reviewed in 1972 by a WHO study group with the significant observation that there was still not enough well substantiated basic information about immunization by this route. The value of the pig as an experimental model for E.coli associated enteritis was highlighted. In this context it is worth noting that the parameters of health used in the studies presently reported, were not considered. Furthermore it is significant that the majority of investigators have been concerned with evaluating oral immunization in mature subjects. In the young unweaned animal, the benefits of enteric immunity may be more dramatically presented for it is growing rapidly at this time and elimination of a growth check over the critical post-weaning period will register significantly along with other health parameters.

References

Allen, W. D. and Porter, P. (1973). The relative distribution of IgM and IgA cells in intestinal mucosa and lymphoid tissue of the young pig and their significance in the ontogenesis of secretory immunity. Immunology, **24,** 493

Allen, W. D. and Porter, P. (1975). The localization of immunoglobulins in intestinal mucosa and the production of secretory antibodies in response to intraluminal administration of bacterial antigens in the pre-ruminant calf. Clin. Exp. Immunol., **21,** 407

Allen, W. D., Smith, C. G. and Porter, P. (1973). Localization of intracellular immunoglobulin A in porcine intestinal mucosa using enzyme labelled antibody. Immunology, **25,** 55

Atkins, A. M., Schofield, G. C. and Reeders, T. (1971). Studies on the structure and distribution of IgA containing cells in the gut of the pig. J. Anat., 109, 385

Brandtzaeg, P. (1974). Mucosal and glandular distribution of immunoglobulin components. Immunology, 26, 1101—1114.

Butler, J. E., Kiddy, C. A., Maxwell, C., Hylton, M. B. and Asofsky, R. (1971). Synthesis of immunoglobulins in various tissues of the cow. J. Dairy Sci., 54, 1324

Cebra, J. J. (1969). Immunoglobulins and immunocytes. Bact. Rev., 33, 151

Eidelman, S. and Davies, S. D. (1968). Immunoglobulin content of intestinal mucosal plasma cells in ataxia telangiectasia. Lancet, i, 884

Freter, R. and Gangarosa, E. J. (1963). Oral Immunization and production of coproantibody in human volunteers. J. Immunol., 91, 724

Lawton, A. R., Asofsky, R., Hylton, M. B. and Cooper, M. D. (1972). Suppression of immunoglobulin synthesis in mice. J. Exp. Med., 135, 277

Mattioli, C. A. and Tomasi, T. B. (1973). The life span of IgA plasma cells from the mouse intestine. J. Exp. Med., 138, 452

Ogra, P. L. and Karzon, D. T. (1969). Distribution of polio virus antibody in serum nasopharynx and alimentary tract following segmental immunization of lower alimentary tract with Polio vaccine. J. Immunol., 102, 1423

Poger, M. E. and Lamm. M. E. (1974). Localization of free and bound secretory component in human intestinal epithelial cells. J. Exp. Med., 139, 629

Porter, P. and Allen, W. D. (1969). Intestinal IgA in the pig. Experientia, 26, 90

Porter, P., Kenworthy, R. and Allen, W. D. (1974). Effect of oral immunization with E.coli antigens on post weaning enteric infection in the young pig. Vet. Rec., 95, 99

Porter, P., Kenworthy, R., Holme, D. W. and Horsefield, S. (1973). E. coli antigens as dietary additives for oral immunization of pigs. Trials with pig creep feeds. Vet. Rec., 92, 630

Porter, P., Kenworthy, R., Noakes, D. E. and Allen, W. D. (1974). Intestinal antibody secretion in the young pig in response to oral immunization with E. coli. Immunology, 27, 841

Porter, P. Kenworthy, R. and Thompson, I. (1975). Oral immunization and its significance in the prophylactic control of enteritis in the preruminant calf. Vet. Rec., **97**, 24

Porter, P. and Noakes, D. E. (1970). Immunoglobulin A in bovine serum and external secretions. Biochim. Biophys. Acta, **214**, 107

Porter, P., Noakes, D. E. and Allen, W. D. (1972). Intestinal secretion of immunoglobulin in the pre-ruminant calf. Immunology, **23**, 299

Roy, J. B. H., Palmer, J., Shillam, K. W. G., Ingram, P. L. and Wood, P. C. (1955). The nutritive value of colostrum for the calf. 10.Relationship between the period of time that a calf house has been occupied and the incidence of scouring and mortality in young calves. Br. J. Nutr., **9**, 11

Smith, J. W. (1960). The ecology of the intestinal bacteria of the calf with particular regard to E. coli. Vet. Rec., **72**, 1178

Smith, H. W. (1962). Observations on the aetiology of neonatal diarrhoea (Scours) in calves. J. Path. Bact., **84**, 147

Stobo, J. D. and Tomasi, T. B. (1966). A low molecular weight immuno-globulin antigenically related to IgM. J. Clin. Invest., **46**, 1329

Swann Report (1969). Joint Committee on the Use of Antibiotics in Animal Husbandry and Veterinary Medicine. H.M.S.O. London.

Vaerman, J. P. (1970). Studies on IgA immunoglobulin in man and animals; Thesis, Université Catholique de Louvain

World Health Organization Technical Report (1972). Oral Enteric Bacterial Vaccines, Serial No. 500

10

Absorption and endogenous production of immunoglobulins in calves

A. J. HUSBAND, M. R. BRANDON and A. K. LASCELLES

INTRODUCTION

There is little or no placental transfer of antibody in ruminants, the young acquiring passive immunity soon after birth by the intestinal absorption of antibody present in the dam's colostrum. Thus, there is an abrupt change in the concentration of antibody or total immunoglobulin in blood serum of newborn ruminants from negligible values at birth to high values soon after ingesting colostrum (cf. Brambell, 1970). Subsequently, the concentration of immunoglobulin in serum declines, due primarily to biological decay of the passively acquired protein, but after some weeks the young, responding to the many antigenic influences to which it is now exposed, begins to synthesize increasing quantities of immunoglobulin. Hence, there must be a period just prior to the onset of endogenous synthesis when immunoglobulin concentration in blood would be at a minimum. It is possible that the concentration of one or more of the classes of immunoglobulins reach such low levels at this time that young ruminants are more susceptible to infectious diseases.

It was in this context that the changes in the concentration of the four immunoglobulins — IgG_1, IgG_2, IgM and IgA — were measured in the blood serum of calves from birth to 18 weeks of age. The primary aims were to determine (a) the efficiency of absorption of immunoglobulin from the intestine of the newborn calf, (b) the relative rates of decline of the individual immunoglobulins in the serum of calves fed known

93

quantities of immunoglobulins, (c) the time of onset of endogenous production of each immunoglobulin and (d) the influence of passively acquired immunoglobulin on endogenous synthesis.

The effect of corticosteroid on these processes was also investigated using newborn unsuckled calves born of cows treated with Opticortenol (dexamethasone trimethylacetate 0.5%, CIBA). Opticortenol is a long-acting synthetic glucocorticoid which is administered to cows to induce premature calving. It is slowly released from its intramuscular depot and crosses the placenta to enter the fetal circulation thus subjecting the fetus to elevated and presumably stable levels of corticosteroid. It is therefore an important practical consideration to know whether this drug affects intestinal closure as well as endogenous immunoglobulin production as has previously been suggested (Smeaton, 1969) and at the same time the model provides an opportunity to study the fundamental question of the effects of this hormone on neonatal immunity.

MATERIALS AND METHODS

Absorption and endogenous production of immunoglobulins in normal calves

Seven newborn unsuckled calves were weighed and a sample of blood taken immediately prior to feeding. They were then each fed 1 litre of their dam's colostrum 2-3 h after birth and 4 h later an additional 1 litre of the same colostrum was fed. They were subsequently fed whole milk until 2 weeks of age and then milk replacer until 8 weeks and were allowed to graze on mixed pasture.

An additional 11 calves were deprived of colostrum. They were separated from their dams before suckling had occurred and were not fed for the first 12 h of life. They were then fed only small amounts of milk until 2 days old, by which time intestinal closure was expected to have occurred. They then received whole milk and were given access to pasture as described for the colostrum fed calves.

Blood samples were collected from all calves at intervals until 18 weeks of age. The concentrations of IgG_1, IgG_2, IgM and IgA in serum, and in the colostral whey of each cow, was determined as described by Brandon, Watson and Lascelles (1971) using the single radial immunodiffusion technique (Mancini, Carbonara and Heremans, 1965).

94

Effect of corticosteroid on absorption and endogenous production of immunoglobulins

Eleven cows were injected intramuscularly with 40 mg Opticortenol in the last 2 months of gestation. At birth calves were removed from their dams before they had suckled, then weighed, and a blood sample was taken. They were then fed 1 litre of mixed colostrum 1-2 h after birth and 4 h later an additional 1 litre from the same colostrum mixture was fed. Three newborn non suckled calves obtained from cows which had undergone a normal gestation were also fed the same quantity of the colostrum in an identical fashion. Whereas plasma samples were collected from all calves for up to 48 h, only 5 of the treated and 2 of the untreated calves were sampled at regular intervals until 18 weeks of age. These calves were reared as for the colostrum fed calves described above.

The plasma volume of the calves was determined by the Evans Blue dye (T-1824) method exactly 12 h after the first feed of colostrum. The concentrations of IgG_1, IgG_2, IgM and IgA were measured in serum and whey samples by single radial immunodiffusion.

Table 1 Concentrations (mg/ml) of immunoglobulins in the serum of pre-suckled calves and in the dam's colostrum

Calf or cow		IgG_1	IgG_2	IgM	IgA
1	S	0.18	0.14	0.12	0.00
	C	54.89	3.85	5.32	1.89
2	S	0.07	0.11	0.00	0.00
	C	32.34	1.37	3.38	1.07
3	S	0.43	0.09	0.23	0.00
	C	28.11	3.08	7.54	1.77
4	S	0.03	0.05	0.08	0.19
	C	70.74	4.98	6.72	11.15
5	S	0.15	0.05	1.70	0.00
	C	40.05	4.37	6.03	3.72
6	S	0.03	0.12	0.00	0.00
	C	66.23	5.53	12.95	9.61
7	S	3.98	0.59	4.67	1.82
	C	45.33	4.66	7.74	3.60

S = Serum
C = Colostrum

95

RESULTS

Absorption and endogenous production of immunoglobulins in normal calves

Immunoglobulins in pre-suckled serum and colostrum

The concentrations of the four immunoglobulins in the pre-suckled serum of the seven calves and in the colostrum subsequently fed to each calf are given in Table 1.

It is evident from these results that no particular immunoglobulin was uniformly predominant in the serum of the pre-suckled calves. IgG_1 and IgG_2 were present in detectable concentrations in the serum of all calves, whereas IgM and IgA were absent from the sera of two and five calves respectively. In calf 4 IgA was present in higher concentrations than the remaining three immunoglobulins, IgM was predominant in calves 5 and 7, IgG_1 in calves 1 and 3, and IgG_2 in calves 2 and 6. The high concentration of all immunoglobulins in calf 7 was particularly striking.

It may be seen from Table 1 that the concentration of the immunoglobulins in colostrum varied considerably between cows. In all cases IgG_1 predominated, its concentration being 2-5 times greater than the sum of the concentrations of the remaining three immunoglobulins.

Table 2 Concentrations of immunoglobulins in blood serum of calves at intervals after birth. Values presented are means (mg/ml) ± SE

Time (days)	IgG_1	IgG_2	IgM	IgA
0	0.70 ± 0.55	0.16 ± 0.07	0.97 ± 0.66	0.29 ± 0.26
½	14.54 ± 2.15	1.96 ± 0.40	6.14 ± 1.20	2.92 ± 0.86
1	16.32 ± 1.51	2.09 ± 0.42	6.01 ± 1.41	2.42 ± 0.85
2	14.43 ± 1.18	1.70 ± 0.30	4.65 ± 1.34	2.02 ± 0.81
4	13.69 ± 1.23	1.38 ± 0.17	3.21 ± 0.91	0.97 ± 0.40
8	12.45 ± 1.25	1.19 ± 0.15	1.68 ± 0.36	0.35 ± 0.10
16	10.43 ± 1.04	1.24 ± 0.11	0.99 ± 0.20	0.04 ± 0.03
32	10.75 ± 1.25	1.49 ± 0.33	0.76 ± 0.17	0.04 ± 0.03
64	12.09 ± 1.20	4.86 ± 0.84	1.47 ± 0.35	0.19 ± 0.03
128	11.88 ± 0.91	4.92 ± 0.57	2.91 ± 0.59	0.21 ± 0.04

Changes in concentrations of immunoglobulins after feeding

The changes in concentrations of immunoglobulin in calf serum with time after feeding are presented in Table 2. The concentrations of all immunoglobulins rose sharply after feeding, IgM and IgA reaching peak levels at the first sampling ($\frac{1}{2}$ day) and IgG_1 and IgG_2 at the second sampling (1 day) after the first feed of colostrum. In accord with its predominance in colostrum, the concentration of IgG_1 in calf serum was substantially higher than any of the other immunoglobulins.

The initial increase in concentration was followed by a decline after which the concentrations stabilized for a period before they began to increase (Table 2). It is evident from the results in Table 2 that the concentrations of IgA and IgM declined almost to zero before beginning to increase again. The results for IgA were particularly striking in this regard, being undetectable in the serum of five calves 16-64 days after feeding.

Apparent efficiency of absorption of immunoglobulins

A measure of the apparent efficiency of absorption of the various immunoglobulins was obtained by computing the ratio (expressed as a percentage) of the quantity estimated to be present in the circulation after

Table 3 Apparent efficiency of absorption

$$\left(\frac{\text{amount of immunoglobulin in circulation}^* \times 100}{\text{amount fed}} \% \right) \text{ of } IgG_1 \ IgG_2,$$

IgA and IgM. Values presented are means $\pm$ SE

	IgG_1	IgG_2	IgA	IgM
Mean	43.9%	58.9%	71.0%	94.7%
Standard error	$\pm$ 4.1%	$\pm$ 10.4%	$\pm$ 14.5%	$\pm$ 9.0%
**Tukey's h.s.d.				

* Pre-feeding value subtracted.
** Means underscored by the same line are not significantly different (p<0.05) according to Tukey's honestly significant difference (h.s.d.) test (cf. Steel and Torrie, 1960)

absorption was complete, to the quantity fed in colostrum. The quantity in plasma was obtained by calculating the product of the peak concentration of each immunoglobulin in the serum (corrected by subtracting the appropriate pre-feeding concentration) and the plasma volume. The latter was taken to be 7.0% of the body weight at birth (see data below for Opticortenol-treated calves). The results of these analyses are presented in Table 3. It may be seen that the magnitude of the ratios decreased in the following order: $IgM > IgA > IgG_2 > IgG_1$. The multiple comparison procedure of Tukey (cf. Steel and Torrie, 1960) was used to determine the significance of the differences between these ratios. It was found that the ratio for IgM was significantly greater ($p < 0.05$) than those for IgG_1 and IgG_2 and no other differences were significant (Table 3).

Pattern of change of the serum concentrations of immunoglobulins

In order to offset the variation in the concentration of the four immunoglobulins in serum attributable to the large differences in the quantities fed in the colostrum, the serum concentrations for each calf were expressed as a percentage of the peak values (values at ½ or 1 day after first feeding) and plotted against $\log_2$ (time). These results are illustrated in Figure 1. All curves were characteristically composed of three components — an initial phase of decline, a phase during which there was little change in concentration followed by a third phase of increasing concentration. The initial phase of these curves appeared to be linear; an analysis of variance revealed highly significant linear components for each immunoglobulin ($p < 0.001$) with deviations from linear regression representing less than 3% of the total variation attributable to time differences (Table 4).

From the orthogonal sums of squares in the above analyses it was possible to calculate the regression coefficients which represented disappearance rates for the four immunoglobulins (Table 5). The significance of the difference between these coefficients was tested using Student's t-test. This showed that the regression coefficients for IgG_1 and IgG_2 were not significantly different, nor were those for IgM and IgA. However, the coefficients for IgG_1 and IgG_2 were significantly less than those for IgM ($p < 0.001$) and IgA ($p < 0.01$) reflecting the more rapid disappearance of IgA and IgM from the circulation.

It is evident that the increase in the concentration of immunoglobulin in the third phase of the curve in Figure 1 was associated with a

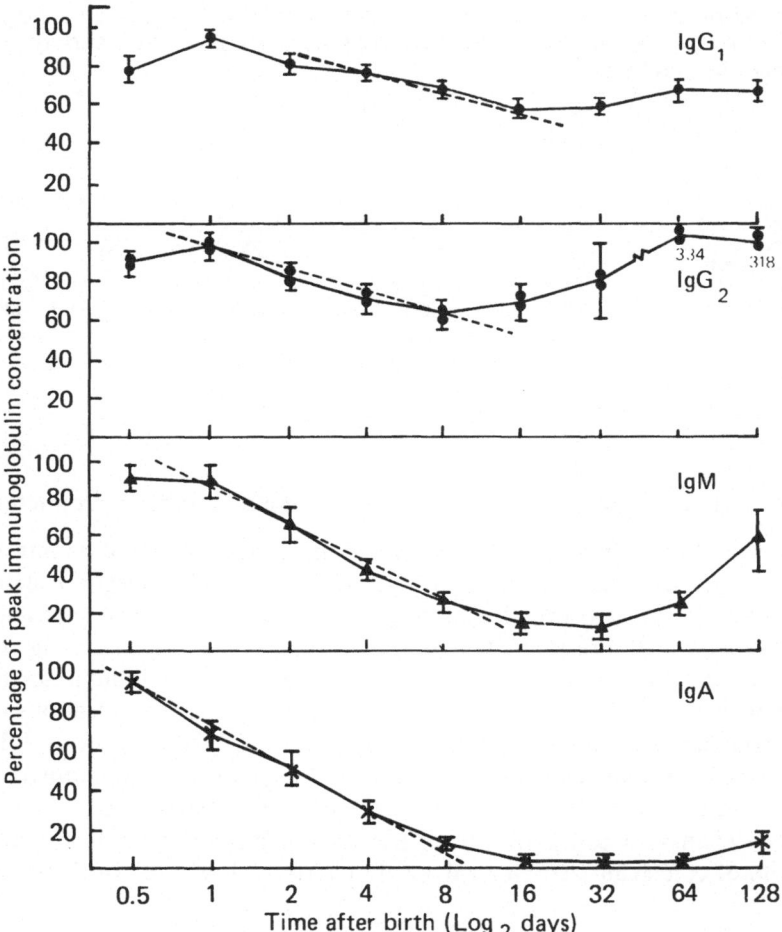

Figure 1 Changes in the serum concentration of IgG_1, IgG_2, IgM and IgA (expressed as a percentage of peak concentration) with time after birth. Plotted points represent means $\pm$ SE

significant endogenous production of immunoglobulin. The results suggest that endogenous production of IgG_1, IgG_2 and IgM actually commenced somewhat earlier, probably at the beginning of the plateau phase (Figure 1). On this basis it is concluded that significant endogenous production of IgG_1, IgG_2 and IgM began 8-16 days after birth and at 64 days for IgA.

Table 4 Summaries of the analyses of variance for the initial period of decline in concentration of the four immunoglobulins with time ($\log_2$) after peak concentrations had been reached. Degrees of freedom are shown in brackets

Source of variation	Mean squares			
	IgG_1	IgG_2	IgM	IgA
Calves	449.5 (6)	432.4 (6)	124.5 (6)	234.8 (6)
Times	1305.6* (4)	1716.4** (3)	4721.8** (3)	7373.1** (4)
Linear	5109.7** (1)	5009.8** (1)	14145.2** (1)	29279.9** (1)
Deviations from linear regression	37.9 (3)	69.6 (2)	10.1 (2)	70.9 (3)
Calves × Times	293.2 (24)	221.1 (18)	426.2 (18)	264.3 (24)

p < 0.01
p < 0.001

Effect of maternal antibody on endogenous immunoglobulin production

It is well documented that the passive administration of large quantities of specific antibody inhibits antibody formation. The question arises whether the passive transfer of large quantities of colostral immuno-globulin, which presumably contain antibodies of a wide range of specificities, inhibits endogenous synthesis of immunoglobulin in the newborn calf. This was investigated by measuring the concentrations of the four immunoglobulins, IgG_1, IgG_2, IgA and IgM in a total of 11 colostrum-deprived calves from birth to 128 days of age and comparing the results with those of colostrum fed calves reported above.

The change in concentration of the various immunoglobulins in the serum of colostrum deprived calves after birth is illustrated in Figure 2.

Table 5 Regression coefficients and standard errors for initial phase of decline of immunoglobulin concentrations in calf serum with time ($\log_2$) after peak concentrations had been reached

	IgG_1	IgG_2	IgM	IgA
Regression coefficient	− 8.54	− 11.96	− 20.10	− 20.45
SE	± 2.05	± 1.78	± 2.47	± 1.94

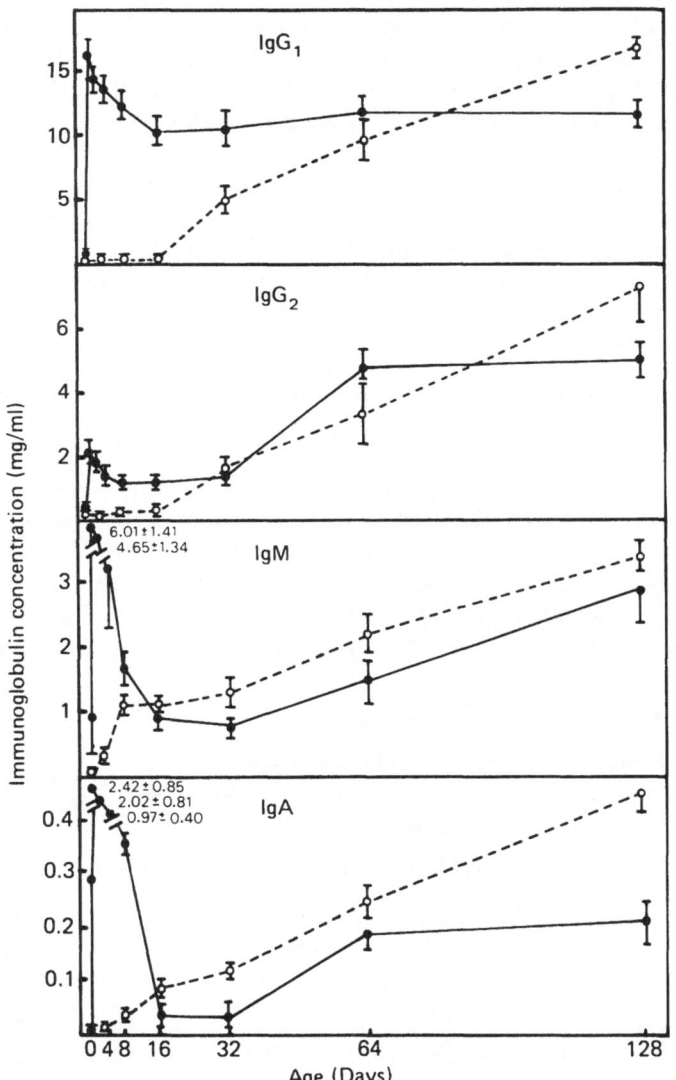

Figure 2 Changes in the serum concentration of IgG_1, IgG , IgM and IgA in colostrum fed (•—•) and colostrum deprived (o---o) calves from birth to 128 days. The data for colostrum fed calves is derived from Table 2.

The concentrations of all immunoglobulins began to increase within a few days of birth and reached quite high levels by 16-32 days. This is in striking contrast to the data for colostrum-fed calves in which it was apparent that endogenous production did not occur until much later than this time; indeed in these calves IgA concentrations almost reached zero between 16 and 32 days (Figures 1 and 2).

It was also apparent from the results that the concentrations of all immunoglobulins at 128 days were higher in the colostrum-deprived calves than the colostrum fed calves. Analysis of the results using Student's t-test revealed that these differences at 128 days were significant for IgG_1 (p < 0.01) and IgA (p < 0.001).

Effect of corticosteroid on absorption and endogenous production

Apparent efficiency of absorption of immunoglobulins

A measure of the apparent efficiency of absorption of the four immunoglobulins was obtained as described above. The mean plasma volume for the 14 calves in this study was determined by T-1824 dilution method to be 6.32 ± 0.15% (mean ± SE) of the body weight. The apparent efficiencies of absorption are presented in Table 6 and it can be seen that the magnitude of the ratios for both treated and untreated

Table 6 Apparent efficiency of absorption

$$\left(\frac{\text{amount of immunoglobulin in circulation* } \times \text{ 100}}{\text{amount fed}} \% \right)$$

of IgG_1, IgG_2, IgA and IgM. Values presented are means ± SE

		IgG_1	IgG	IgA	IgM
Opticortenol-treated calves	Mean	23.4%	29.4%	33.1%	36.4%
	SE	± 3.5%	± 3.8%	± 4.5%	± 7.2%
Untreated calves	Mean	45.9%	47.8%	56.6%	87.1%
	SE	± 3.9%	± 1.9%	± 5.7%	±18.0%

* Pre-feeding value subtracted.

Table 7 Concentrations of immunoglobulins in blood serum of Opticortenol-treated and untreated calves at intervals after birth. Values presented are means (mg/ml) ± SE

	Time (days)	IgG_1	IgG_2	IgM	IgA
Opticortenol-treated calves	0	0.06 ± 0.02	0.06 ± 0.02	0.13 ± 0.03	0.02 ± 0.01
	1	3.58 ± 0.93	0.74 ± 0.12	0.70 ± 0.12	0.44 ± 0.17
	8	3.28 ± 0.80	0.67 ± 0.11	0.64 ± 0.14	0.01 ± 0.01
	16	3.25 ± 0.70	0.42 ± 0.01	1.00 ± 0.80	0.01 ± 0.01
	32	8.37 ± 3.25	2.73 ± 1.10	0.87 ± 0.28	0.01 ± 0.01
	64	10.51 ± 2.92	5.05 ± 1.56	1.30 ± 0.33	0.02 ± 0.01
	96	13.94 ± 1.99	6.11 ± 1.33	1.90 ± 0.36	0.14 ± 0.07
	128	14.39 ± 2.12	5.90 ± 0.80	2.34 ± 0.37	0.15 ± 0.08
Untreated calves	0	0.10 ± 0.03	0.09 ± 0.01	0.12 ± 0.06	0.01 ± 0.01
	1	6.40 ± 2.63	1.14 ± 0.48	1.22 ± 0.62	0.58 ± 0.26
	8	4.53 ± 2.71	1.07 ± 0.63	0.45 ± 0.12	0.02 ± 0.02
	16	6.45 ± 4.44	0.86 ± 0.50	0.46 ± 0.13	0.03 ± 0.02
	32	4.50 ± 2.08	0.98 ± 0.41	0.84 ± 0.43	0.10 ± 0.03
	64	7.32 ± 2.04	2.17 ± 0.28	1.40 ± 0.54	0.39 ± 0.07
	96	11.34 ± 1.90	2.37 ± 0.07	1.66 ± 0.77	0.32 ± 0.03
	128	13.20 ± 2.73	6.11 ± 0.55	1.82 ± 0.22	0.35 ± 0.06

calves decreases in the order: $IgM > IgA > IgG_2 > IgG_1$. Analysis of these data by Student's t-test (Steel and Torrie, 1960) showed that the ratios for untreated calves were significantly greater ($p < 0.01$) than those for treated calves.

Endogenous production of immunoglobulin

The changes in concentration of immunoglobulin in the serum of treated and untreated calves are presented in Table 7. The concentration of all immunoglobulins rose rapidly after feeding, maximum concentrations 24 h after birth being approx. twice as high for untreated as for treated calves. The time of onset of endogenous production of IgG_1, IgG_2 and IgM for calves treated with Opticortenol was similar to that for the three untreated calves in the present experiment and for the seven colostrum-fed calves in the preceding section. In contrast to the results for the above immunoglobulins, concentrations of IgA in serum of Opticortenol treated calves did not begin to increase until at least 32 days later than for untreated calves (Table 7).

DISCUSSION

The results presented in Table 1 demonstrate the marked hypogamma-globulinaemic state of the calves at birth, although some calves, particularly calf 7, had appreciably higher levels of immunoglobulin than others. The marked difference in the proportion of the four immunoglobulins in the pre-suckled serum of calf 7 compared with those in the dam's colostrum (Table 1) and in the blood of adult cattle (Brandon et al., 1971) militates against the possibilities that the immunoglobulin originated from either colostrum or maternal blood. It is suggested that most of the immunoglobulin in the serum of calf 7 had been synthesized endogenously under the influence of antigens, possibly an infectious agent, transmitted to the fetus by way of the placenta. This is further borne out by the persistence of IgA in detectable concentrations in the sera of the two calves which had significant concentrations of IgA in their pre-suckled sera.

In a study on the quantitative absorption of immunoglobulins by way of the thoracic duct lymph of newborn calves, Brandon and Lascelles (1971) demonstrated conclusively that the efficiency and rate of absorption of all four immunoglobulins from the intestine were similar. Thus, the greater apparent efficiency of absorption of the higher molecular weight IgM (and IgA) compared with IgG (Table 3) suggests that a higher proportion of IgG than IgM had left the bloodstream and entered the interstitial fluid resulting in a gross underestimate of the quantity of IgG absorbed. This observation is important in relation to estimates of efficiency of absorption of the various immunoglobulins reported by other workers who have based their calculations on the concentration in calf serum relative to the amount fed (e.g. Klaus, Bennett and Jones, 1969).

IgM was absorbed with an efficiency of 95%. However this is probably an underestimate since some IgM would have been lost from the intravascular compartment — by transfer into the interstitial fluid and biological degradation — during the 12 h period after first feeding. It is suggested therefore that IgM is absorbed with an efficiency approaching 100%. From the results of Brandon and Lascelles (1971) it follows that all immunoglobulins are absorbed at the same high efficiency. The different rates of equilibration of the larger and smaller molecular weight immunoglobulins between blood and interstitial fluid probably also account for the finding that IgG_1 and IgG_2 reach peak concentrations later than IgA and IgM.

104

It seems reasonable to assume, at least in six of the seven calves, that endogenous production was not making a significant contribution to total plasma immunoglobulin during the first 1-2 weeks after birth. Thus it is considered that the initial phase of decline in concentration of the immunoglobulins, which was shown to be linear when plotted against $\log_2$ (time), represented biological decay of the passively transferred immunoglobulin. The calculated regression coefficients revealed that IgM and IgA were degraded more rapidly than IgG_1 and IgG_2. Estimates of the half lives of the various immunoglobulins calculated from the regression curves were 16-32 days for IgG_1 and IgG_2 4 days for IgM and 2.5 days for secretory IgA. These estimates are similar to those for comparable immunoglobulins for the newborn pig reported by Curtis and Bourne (1971).

From the results in Figure 1 and Table 2 it is evident that the concentration of the immunoglobulins in calf serum was minimal between 8 and 32 days after birth and it is reasonable to suggest that calves receiving inadequate quantities of immunoglobulin in their dams' colostrum would be seriously hypogammaglobulinaemic at this time. The question arises as to whether the low concentrations of IgG_2, IgM and IgA during this phase of life, even in calves fed adequate levels of colostral immunoglobulins, is associated with increased susceptibility to certain diseases. IgA was particularly striking in this regard as in 5 of the 7 calves the concentration was zero during the period 16-64 days after birth.

With respect to the effect of maternal antibody on endogenous immunoglobulin synthesis the results demonstrate that this occurred much earlier in colostrum deprived calves than colostrum fed calves (Figure 2) and indeed the serum concentration of IgG_1 and IgA at 128 days in colostrum deprived calves exceeded those for the fed calves. This appears to reflect a feedback inhibition mechanism.

It can be seen from Figure 2 that the difference in endogenous production of immunoglobulin between colostrum deprived and colostrum fed calves was most striking in the case of IgA. In this connection, it is recalled that most serum IgA is derived from the gut-associated lymphoid tissue (Beh, Watson and Lascelles, 1974) and as this is the region where the highest concentration of passively acquired maternal antibody occurs following ingestion and absorption of colostrum, it is suggested that this initial saturation causes antibody feedback inhibition of IgA production in this area. Thus it would appear that the delay in endogenous immunoglobulin production in colostrum-fed calves (especially for IgA) is a consequence of the effect of maternal antibody rather than immaturity of the lymphoid system.

Opticortenol treatment of cows to induce parturition had a significant effect on absorption and endogenous production of immunoglobulins in the calf. Perhaps the most dramatic consequence was that it reduced the efficiency of absorption of IgM by approximately half that observed in untreated calves and substantial decreases in the apparent efficiencies of absorption were also observed for the remaining immunoglobulins. In accord with these results, Gillette and Filkins (1966) reported that puppies from bitches treated with ACTH or hydrocortisone during the 24 h before birth absorbed colostral immunoglobulin less efficiently.

Opticortenol treatment appeared to have no effect on the time of onset or the magnitude of endogenous synthesis of IgG_1, IgG_2 and IgM. However, it is evident from the results that Opticortenol treatment is responsible for a delay in the endogenous synthesis of IgA. Since virtually all the IgA in serum in ruminants is derived from plasma cells in the lamina propria of the intestine (Beh et al., 1974) it is suggested that Opticortenol either specifically inhibits the development of IgA precursor cells in Peyer's patches (Craig and Cebra, 1971) or depletes the cortisone sensitive helper T-cell population which is known to be essential for normal IgA antibody responses (Clough, Mims and Strober, 1971).

The results of the experiments using Opticortenol suggest that corticosteroids may be implicated in the phenomenon of closure of intestinal absorption of colostral immunoglobulin and in animals undergoing a normal birth the endogenous corticosteroids produced during birth could be directly or indirectly involved in this process. But from a more practical consideration it appears that the use of corticosteroids to induce parturition will place the calf at a serious disadvantage, its health being jeopardized by the disturbances caused to immunoglobulin absorption and synthesis.

References*

Beh, K. J., Watson, D. L. and Lascelles, A. K. (1974). Aust. J. Exp. Biol. Med. Sci., **52**, 81

Brambell, F. W. R. (1970). Frontiers of Biology, Vol. 18, A. Newberger and E. L. Tatum (eds.). (Amsterdam: North-Holland Publishing Company)

Brandon, M. R. and Lascelles, A. K. (1971). Aust. J. Exp. Biol. Med. Sci., **49**, 629

Brandon, M. R., Watson, D. L. and Lascelles, A. K. (1971). Aust. J. Exp. Biol. Med. Sci., **49**, 613

Clough, J. D., Mims, L. H. and Strober, W. (1971). J. Immunol., **106**, 1624

Craig, S. W. and Cebra, J. J. (1971). J. Exp. Med., **134**, 188

Curtis, J. and Bourne, F. J. (1971). Biochim. Biophys. Acta, **236**, 319

Gillette, D D. and Filkins, M. (1966). Am. J. Physiol., **210**, 419

Klaus, G. G. B., Bennett, A. and Jones, E. W. (1969). Immunology, **16**, 235

Mancini, G., Carbonara, A. O. and Heremans, J. F. (1965). Immunochemistry, **2**, 235

Smeaton, T. C. (1969). Gamma-globulin metabolism in lambs. Ph.D. Thesis, Australian National University, Canberra, Australia

Steel, R. G. D. and Torrie, J. H. (1960). Principles and Procedures of Statistics. P.72. (New York: McGraw-Hill Book Co., Inc.)

*FOOTNOTE

Part of the data contained in this chapter has appeared in the following additional publications:

Husband, A. J., Brandon, M. R. and Lascelles, A. K. (1972). Aust. J. Exp. Biol. Med. Sci., **50**, 491

Husband, A. J., Brandon, M. R. and Lascelles, A. K. (1973). Aust. J. Exp. Biol. Med. Sci., **51**, 707

Husband, A. J. and Lascelles, A. K. (1975). Res. Vet. Sci., **18**, 201
Sci., **50**, 491

11

Antigen uptake in the small intestine of guinea pigs infected with Trichinella spiralis

D. I. PRITCHARD, D. CATTY and J. J. HANKES

INTRODUCTION

In nematode infections of the intestine the host is exposed to a complex mixture of antigens released during developmental and reproductive phases of the parasites' life cycles. Antigenic metabolites are released, or secreted actively by the worms, often in very large amounts; they may be released in the lumen of the gut or, in cases where worms invade the epithelial or deeper tissues, they may be deposited in closer association with the reticuloendothelial system of the host. In any event one result of gastrointestinal infestation is an immune response measurable both within the local gut lymphoid tissues and in the general circulation, so it is quite clear that parasite antigens always find their way across the epithelial barrier of the intestine and into the lymphoid tissue, even if no damage to the host is apparent. This subject has been extensively reviewed in recent years (see eg. Dobson, 1972; Catty, 1975a).

In this paper we describe some experiments in which the uptake and transport of metabolic antigens of Trichinella spiralis has been studied, by immunofluorescence, within the tissues of the small intestine of the guinea pig. Although the adult female worms eventually become deeply embedded, by the oral end, within the villi, release of antigens occurs predominantly in the preceding developmental phase (Catty, 1969, 1975b), when infective larvae, more loosely applied to the mucosal surface, undergo a series of moults, growth and differentiation. It is the

109

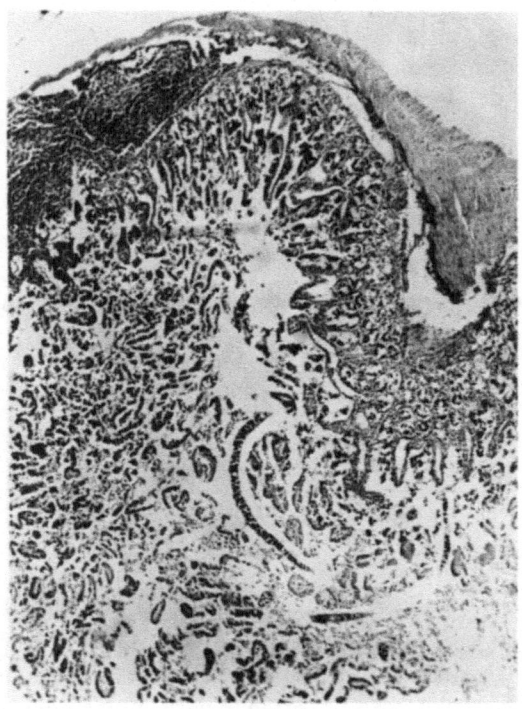

Figure 1 Transverse section of rabbit small intestine infected with a mature adult female Trichinella spiralis in which the worm is cut longitudinally. Developing embryos can be seen within the uterus

uptake of antigens released at this early phase of infection which we have studied.

Life cycle of the parasite

The infective stage consists of larvae encapsulated in the muscles of the host. These are poised for rapid development to adults once the capsules are digested away in the stomach of the new host. The capsules can also be removed in vitro by exposure of chopped, infected meat to pepsin-HCI. The larvae released in the gut pass through moulting and maturation to become adults in about 4 days. In the guinea pig this occurs in the absorptive distal segment of the small intestine. Gravid females can be found at about 6 days, full of developing embryos,

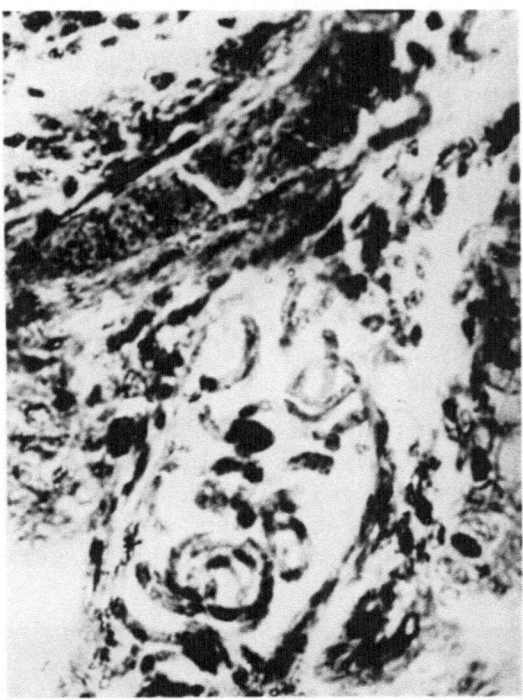

Figure 2 Transverse section of guinea pig jejunum showing the anterior portion of an adult female Trichinella embedded within the submucosa, and beneath, a section of the uterus of the same worm containing embryos. The invasive stage is accompanied by a mixed cell inflammatory reaction.

embedded in the mucosa (Figures 1 and 2). These females release large numbers of small migratory larvae directly into the sub-epithelial tissues and these find their way into the host musculature.

Parasite antigens

In vitro studies using antisera raised by infection and by immunization with metabolites have shown that Trichinella contains a complex group of antigens (Olson, Richards and Ewert, 1960; Tanner and Gregory, 1961; Tanner, 1963). Five or six metabolic antigens, associated with moulting and maturation, are released normally within the intestine in the pre-invasive stage (Mills and Kent, 1965; Catty, 1969). These are the antigens to which the early antibody response is directed and to which antisera can be raised by immunization of rabbits with larval culture supernates. Of these antigens, one is outstanding in its potency as an immunogen. It is a glycoprotein with a molecular weight of 12 000 and is a strong allergen for induction of IgE antibodies and immediate hypersensitivity (Perrudet-Badoux and Binaghi, 1974). From selective immunizations it is known to be a soluble product, probably a secretion released from the oral opening of the worm. The antiserum used in our fluorescence study is directed largely towards this antigen.

METHODS

Fluorescence technique

Guinea pigs were infected with 1000-2000 living larvae by stomach intubation. From 2-15 days after infection the distal segment of the small intestine was snap-frozen in a liquid nitrogen/isopentane mixture and sectioned on a cryostat, or fixed and sectioned for histology. The frozen sections were stained directly with fluorescein-conjugated

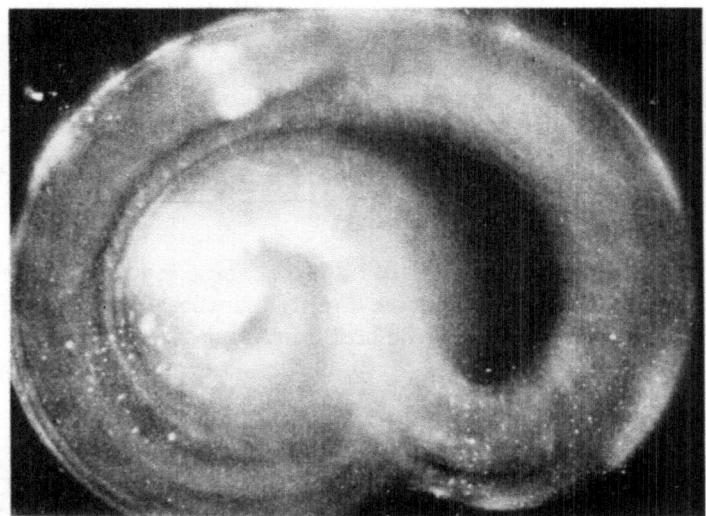

Figure 3 Specific staining of a living Trichinella larva in vitro caused by precipitation of labelled antibody with secreted antigenic metabolites to form an 'oral cap' of fluorescence. Some of this precipitate, loosened from the cap, is also adherent to the cuticle of the worm.

antibody to the larval metabolites. This antibody had been prepared by salt precipitation and DEAE-cellulose fractionation and was a pure IgG preparation. Purification was found to be a necessary step in removal of elements giving non specific staining of the tissues. In addition the labelled IgG was rigorously absorbed with an insoluble preparation of guinea pig intestinal homogenate. Labelled normal rabbit IgG and labelled antibody absorbed with antigen were used as control preparations.

Specificity of labelling

The labelled antibody produced no staining of sections of normal guinea pig intestine. Autofluorescence of gut contents, and of granulocytes strung along the sub-epithelial components of the villi, was apparent.

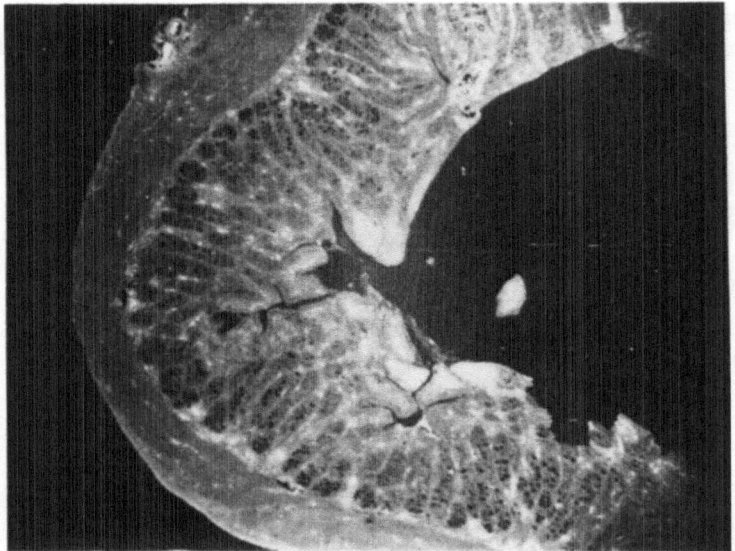

Figure 4 Transverse section of guinea pig jejunum infected with Trichinella for three days and stained with labelled antibody to worm metabolites. Sections of the posterior part of a worm can be seen lying between villi in the upper centre, but the majority of antigen has been released by the oral end of the worm which was situated adjacent to the villi in the centre. The villi in this region are full of cells containing antigen, but some antigen has been carried to the crypt region and even to the blood vessels of the muscularis mucosa (upper left).

113

The granulocytes gave a yellow/red fluorescence, however, easily distinguisable from specific staining. The labelled antibodies stained actively metabolizing larvae maintained in vitro — this showed as an 'oral cap' of immune precipitate formed as the larvae released from the oral opening the metabolic antigens to which the antibody is specific (Figure 3). Dead, non-metabolizing larvae failed to stain in this way.

RESULTS

Pattern of labelling in the infected intestine

Before describing the uptake of antigen it is as well to stress the relationship of the worm to the gut mucosa in the infection stage under study, and the arrangement of the absorptive tissues in the locally infected region. Before maturation of the female, in the first 6 days or so, the developing worms lie loosely between the villi with no evidence of penetration of the epithelium. In primary infections this phase is accompanied by little obvious inflammatory reaction on the part of the

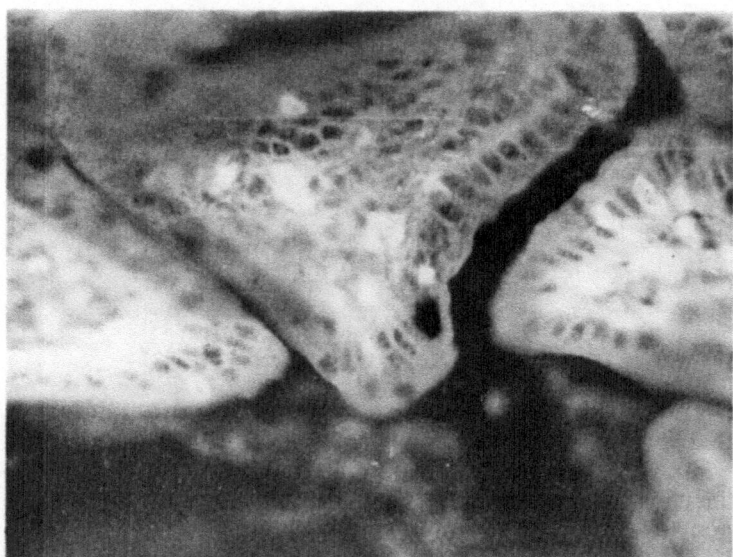

Figure 5 High power of central part of Figure 4, showing tips of villi adjacent to a developing Trichinella larva prior to sectioning. Larval antigen has been taken up by cells within the epithelium and antigen-packed cells fill the tips of the villi.

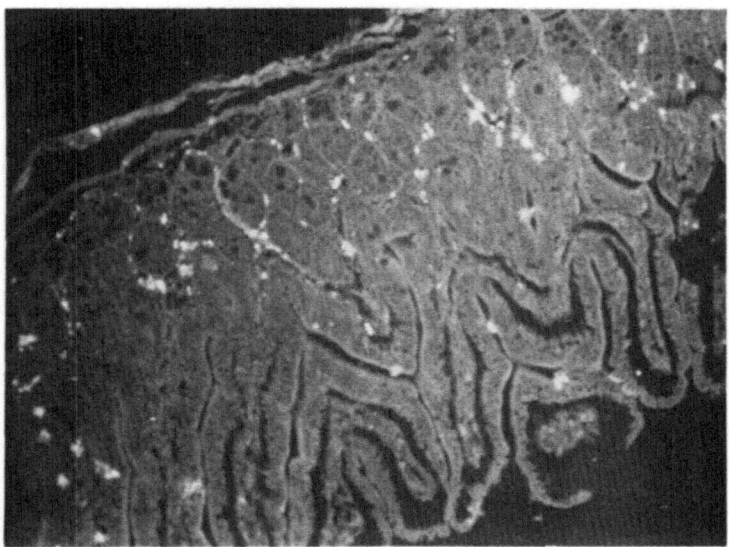

Figure 6 As Figure 4, but the section is not closely associated with a developing larva. Wandering cells in the crypt region, some with dendritic process, can be seen labelled with antigen.

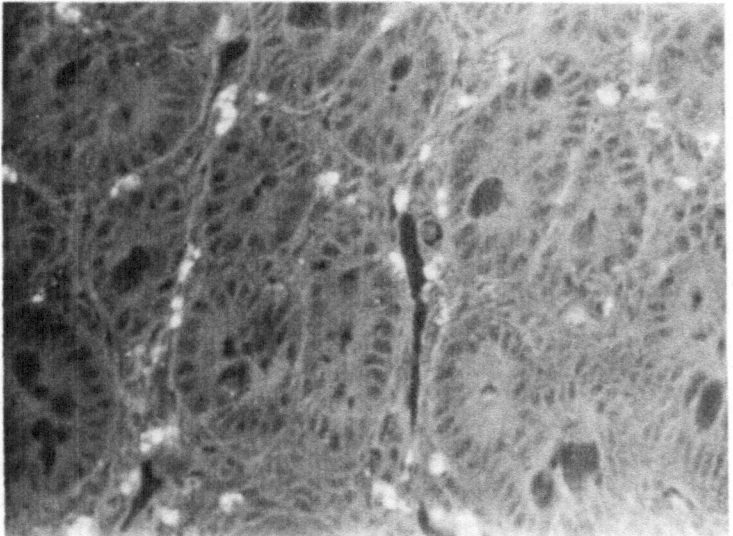

Figure 7 High power part of section shown in Figure 6 in the crypt region, showing the distribution of antigen-containing cells.

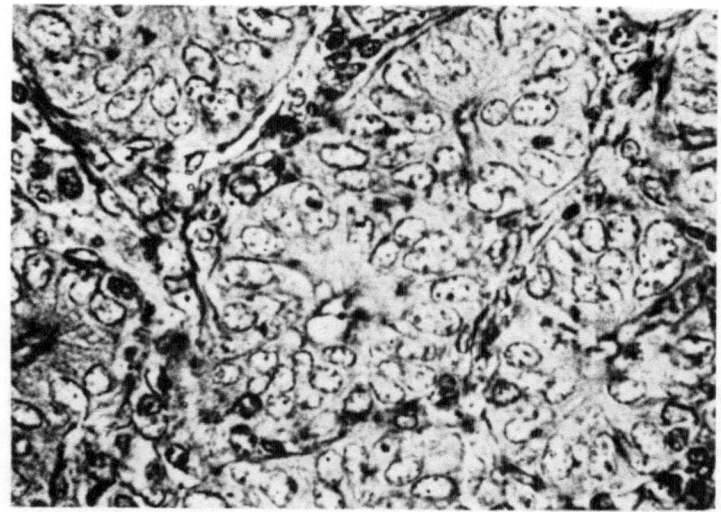

Figure 8 Histological section of the crypt region of guinea pig ileum infected with Trichinella for 10 days. A mixed cell infiltrate can be identified between the bases of villi. Cells labelling for antigen, as shown in Figure 7, are present within this population.

host. The villi, in the absorptive region of the small intestine, have a border of columnar epithelial cells coated with mucous, and an internal mixed cell population of lymphoid cells, granulocytes, histiocytes and others.

How do the parasite metabolic antigens find their way across this barrier? Antigens released in the first few days of development of the larvae can be seen to be taken up by the intestinal tissues. In Figure 4 the position of a worm can be clearly seen by the high concentration of antigen close to the epithelial border. One can observe that some antigen has already reached the blood vessels in the muscularis mucosa and is also widely distributed within the intestinal tissues, within the core of the villi closest to the worms and at the bases of the villi in the crypt region. At higher power (Figure 5) it becomes evident that the antigen is not diffusing between cells in the extra-cellular fluid, but is being taken up actively and transported inwards by what seems to be an active cell migration process. At sites not closely associated with a parasite the antigen is seen in dendritic type cells lying at the bases of the crypts (Figures 6 and 7). These may not be of the same type as those seen taking up antigen at the epithelium, but have the appearance of phagocytes,

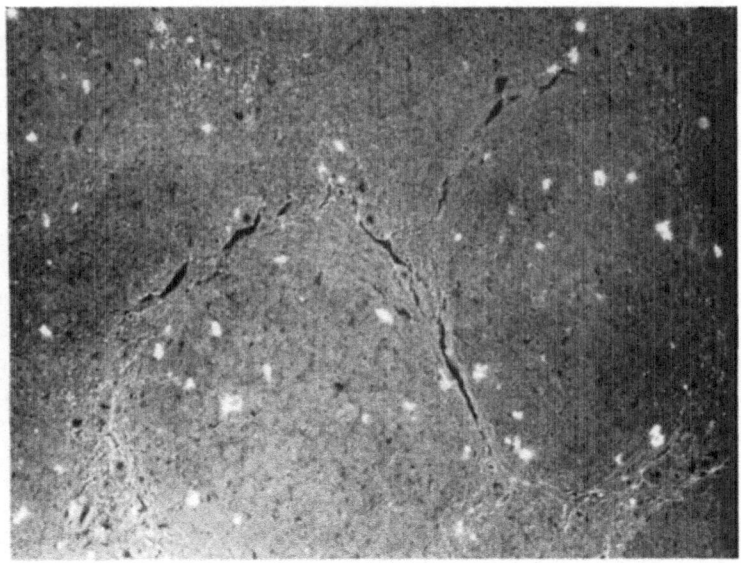

Figure 9 Section of Peyer's patch at low magnification from 3 day infected guinea pig proximal ileum showing dendritic cells within the lymphoid lobules staining strongly for larval metabolite antigens

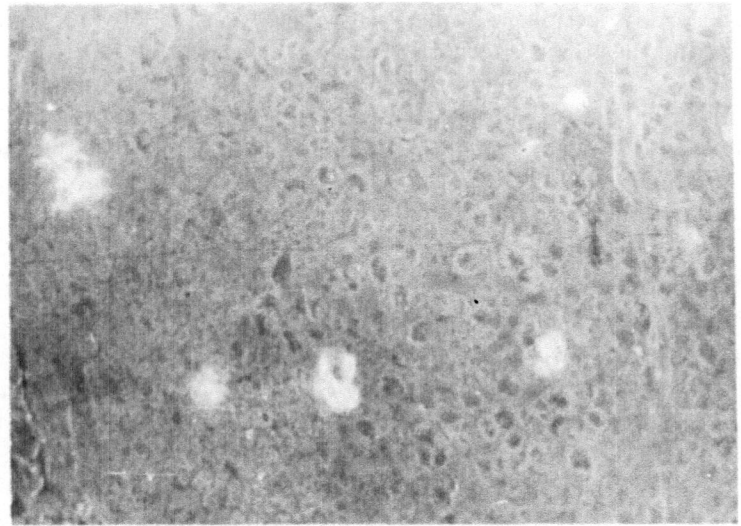

Figure 10 High magnification of Figure 9 showing part of one lobule with several antigen containing dendritic cells clearly identifiable

117

some with very obvious dendritic processes. Such cells reach peak numbers about 10 days after infection at which time they can be seen in the crypt region as part of a mixed cell inflammation (Figure 8).

The organized lymphoid tissue of the small intestine consists of Peyer's patches — large accumulations of lymphocytes arranged in lobules of tissue placed between the muscularis mucosa and the villous region. Antigen-positive dendritic cells appear in the Peyer's patches within 3 days of infection (Figures 9 and 10). The route by which such cells gain access to the lymphoid tissue is not known but they do not appear to migrate directly across the lamina propria and probably arrive via small blood vessels or lymphatics if these exist. The role of Peyer's patch lymphocytes in the subsequent local antibody response of the infected intestine is also somewhat of a mystery. No antibody producing cells are seen in the Peyer's patches, although clearly antigen reaches this tissue.

CONCLUSION

We have shown that the major antigenic components of the metabolites of this intestinal nematode parasite are taken up by the absorptive region of the intestine during a period prior to parasite penetration of the tissues. The uptake is, at least in part, an active process, with epithelial cells and perhaps macrophages involved. The relationship between cells at the absorptive periphery of the gut which are seen to take up antigen actively, and the cells, also with antigen in the cytoplasm, which migrate through the tissues, remains to be explored. The 'macrophage' or dendritic cell appears to be active in carrying the antigen away from the site of parasite/host contact and some antigen reaches the local lymphoid tissues in this way. No evidence was seen of passive diffusion of antigen within the intracellular spaces of the intestinal tissues.

References

Catty, D. (1969). The immunology of nematode infections: trichinosis in guinea pigs as a model. Monogr. Allergy, Vol. 5. (Basel: S. Karger)

Catty, D. (1975a). Immune responses to gastrointestinal infestations (Protozoa and Nematodes). In: (P. Asquith, (ed.), Immunology of the Gastrointestinal Tract. (London: Churchill Livingstone)

Catty, D. (1975b). Immunity and acquired resistance to trichinosis. In: (S. Cohen and E. Sadun, (eds.), The Immunology of Parasitic Infections. (Oxford: Blackwell Scientific Publications)

Dobson, C. (1972). Immune response to gastrointestinal helminths. In:

(E. J. L. Soulsby, (ed.), Immunity to Animal Parasites, pp. 191-222. (New York: Academic Press)

Mills, C. K. and Kent, N. H. (1965). Excretions and secretions of Trichinella spiralis and their role in immunity. Exp. Parasit., **16**, 300

Olson, L. J., Richards, B. and Ewert, A. (1960). Detection of metabolic antigens from nematode larvae by a microculture-agar gel technique. Tex. Rep. Biol. Med., **18**, 254

Tanner, C. E. (1963). Immunochemistry of the antigens of Trichinella spiralis larvae. II. Some physico-chemical properties of these antigens. Exp. Parasit., **14**, 337

Tanner, C. E. and Gregory, J. (1961). Immunochemistry of the antigens of Trichinella spiralis larvae. I. Identification and enumeration of antigens. Canad. J. Microbiol., **7**, 473

Perrudet-Badoux, A. and Binaghi, R. A. (1974). Isolation and properties of a soluble antigen of Trichinella spiralis. Immunology, **26**, 1217

12

Antibody production in the intestine-associated immune tissues following antigen stimulation in the bowel lumen

R. V. HEATLEY and J. M. STARK

INTRODUCTION

Many patients suffering from chronic inflammatory disorders of the gastrointestinal tract, and also some normal people, have circulating antibodies to both food protein and intestinal bacterial antigens. It is therefore apparent that immunogenic molecules can penetrate the gastrointestinal mucosa.

We have been studying the circumstances in which antigens in the intestinal lumen of experimental animals may initiate a systemic antibody response and to what degree antigen absorption from the gastrointestinal tract is important in the initiation of this response. We have also attempted to identify the site of production of these antibodies in response to intestinal antigenic stimulation.

The work we are going to describe was performed using the rat as the experimental animal model. The antigens were all administered by injection at laparotomy into the intestinal lumen. Antibody responses were measured by a modified Farr ammonium sulphate precipitation technique (Mitchison, 1971).

121

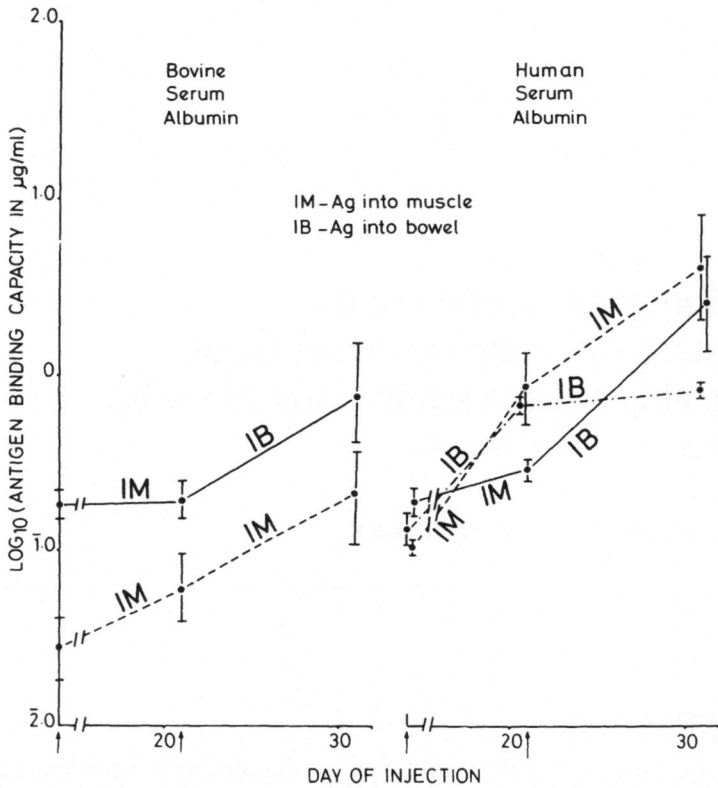

Figure 1 Rat antibody responses to bovine and human serum albumin. The antigen was given intramuscularly (I.M.) or into the bowel lumen (IB). Each point is the mean response of five animals ± standard error. The primary dose intramuscularly was 1 mg, the secondary dose 100 μg. The intrabowel doses were 10 × greater.

SELECTION OF ANTIGEN

We first chose to study the systemic antibody response to bovine serum albumin (BSA), given both intramuscularly (i.m.) and into the bowel, since this has previously been used successfully by several other investigators. However, we found BSA to be a poor immunogen when given both i.m. and into the bowel (Figure 1), sensitization being inconsistent. We then used human serum albumin (HSA), and found this to give more consistent results both intramuscularly and also into the bowel lumen, even when the bowel route was used for initial sensitization

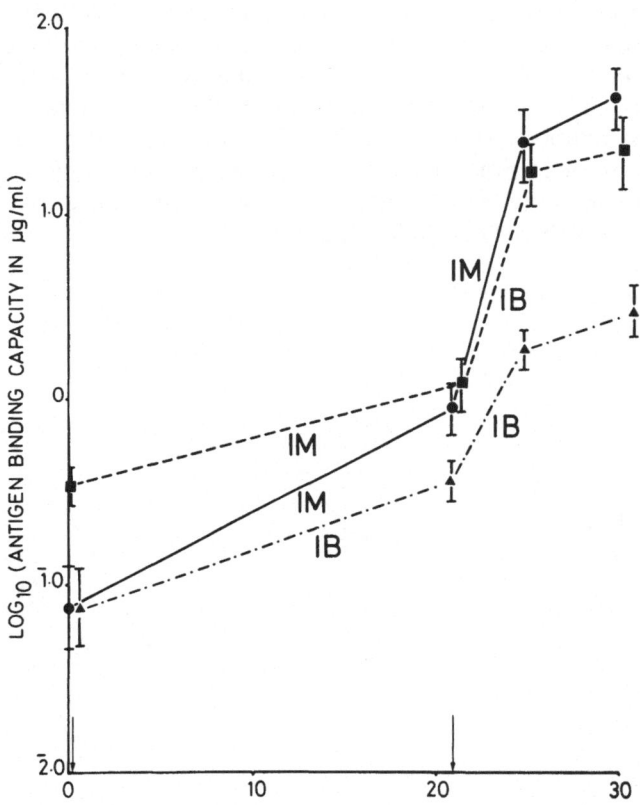

Figure 2 Rat antibody responses to diphtheria toxoid. The primary dose intramuscularly was 40 μg, the secondary 10 μg. The intrabowel doses were 10 × greater. Intramuscular antigen for primary and secondary stimulation (•). Intramuscular primary and intrabowel secondary (■). Intrabowel route for both (▲).

(Figure 1). Following this we studied diphtheria toxoid, and found this to be a fairly potent antigen giving consistent and reproducible results when given into the intestinal lumen (Figure 2). In all these experiments the intrabowel dose of antigen was ten times the dose given intramuscularly in the parallel experiment.

We became interested at that time in a modified antigen studied by Coon and Hunter (1973). They reported that when BSA was heavily conjugated with a simple lipid (C_{12} fatty acid), no detectable antibody

123

was induced by this antigen, but a marked delayed type hypersensitivity response was obtained. We decided to study this conjugate in the bowel lumen, but chose to acylate HSA, since this albumin in our experience was the better stimulator of antibody synthesis in the bowel.

When this acylated HSA was used in the bowel lumen a greatly enhanced antibody response resulted (Heatley and Stark, 1975). The response varied with the degree of acylation, the optimal response (comparable to that with incomplete Freund's adjuvant with 1 mg HSA i.m.) being with 22% acylation (Figure 3).

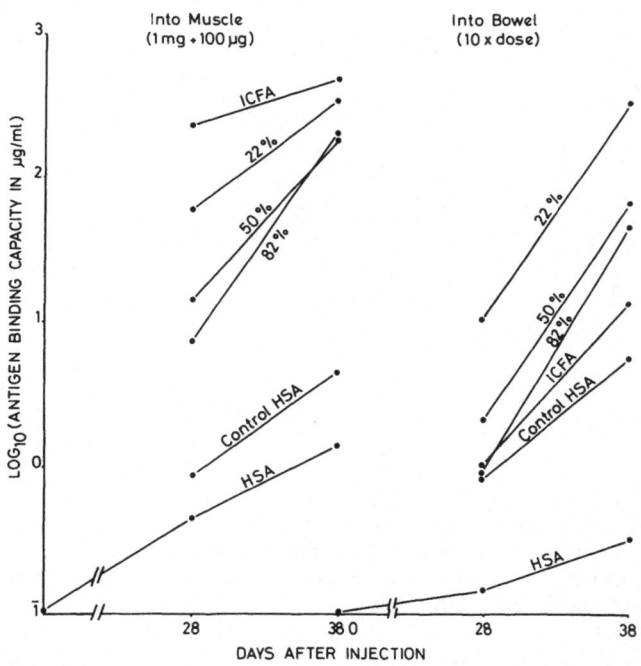

Figure 3 Rat antibody responses to human serum albumin (HSA). The effect of increased acylation (quoted as percentage) on the immunogenicity of HSA when given (a) intramuscularly (1 mg + 100 μg) or (b) into the bowel lumen (10 mg + 1 mg). Each point represents the mean log 10 antigen binding capacity for five animals when tested at 1 μg/ml. Control HSA = albumin exposed to solvent mixtures only without acylating agent. (From Heatley and Stark, Immunology, **29**, 143, 1975, by permission of the Editor and Blackwell Scientific Publications)

FEATURES OF SELECTED ANTIGEN

Having recognized an antigen which was potent when given into the bowel lumen and being able to modify the response by altering the degree of acylation we examined various properties of these conjugates in an attempt to explain the enhanced immunogenicity.

Physical characteristics

The degree of molecular aggregation and the adhesiveness of the antigenic molecules would influence their interaction with the surface cells of the gut, their transfer across the mucosa, and their subsequent handling in the submucosal layers.

The degree of molecular aggregation of lipid conjugated HSA (LCHSA) molecules was determined by passage through a Sephadex

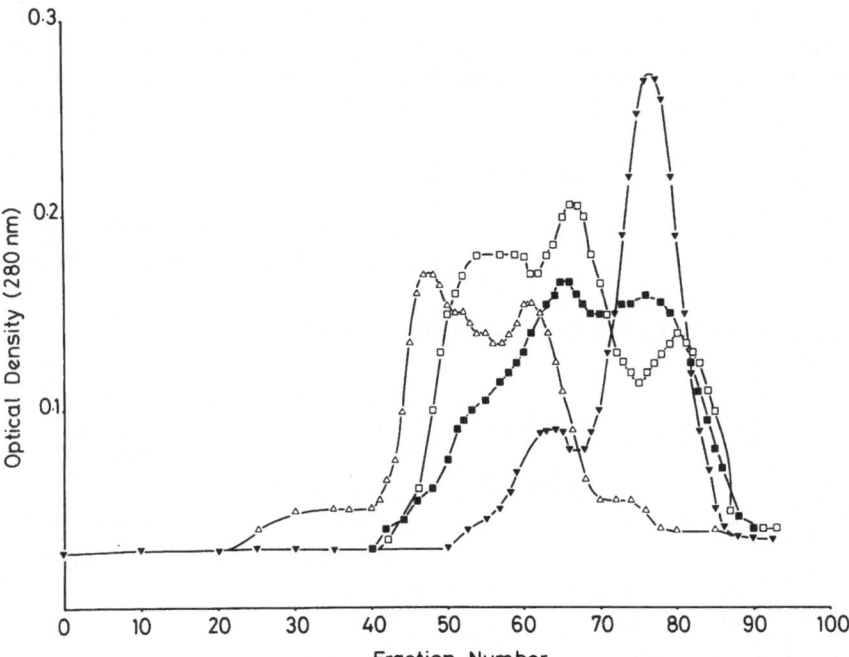

Figure 4 Sephadex G-200 gel filtration of acylated human serum albumin preparations (each approx. 30 mg) in a 2.5 × 90 cm column. Human serum albumin (HSA) (▼). Percentage acylation of HSA: 30 (■); 75 (□); 90 (△). (From Heatley and Stark, Immunology, **29**, 143, 1975, by permission of the Editor and Blackwell Scientific Publications)

G-200 column. Protein with 30% of its epsilon amino groups acylated shows a reduction of monomeric and increase in dimeric and other low polymeric species when compared with HSA itself. The degree of polymerization is more obvious with higher acylations (Figure 4).

In an attempt to assess the degree to which LCHSA would adhere to cells, suspensions of rat peritoneal cells were incubated for one hour at 37 °C with ratio iodinated protein antigens at three different concentrations. After the cells had been washed three times, significantly higher amounts of the acylated proteins remained attached to the peritoneal cells (Table 1) (p $<$ 0.001 for 1 μg/ml). The percentage attachment increased with acylation.

Because of their adhesiveness, the lipidated HSA molecules will tend to remain in the gut wall and initiate antibody formation there, rather than enter the lymphatics or portal venous system. The tendency of LCHSA to aggregate and attach to cell surfaces would be likely to confer an immunogenic advantage not only because aggregates of protein immunogens are immunogenic, rather than tolerogenic (Frei, 1964), but also since macrophage attached protein is more immunogenic than protein in free solution (Spitznagel and Allison, 1970).

Effect of acylation on lymphatic absorption

The routes available for transport of antigen from the gut are the portal vein through the liver to the systemic circulation, or by the mesenteric

Table 1 Attachment of radiolabelled proteins to rat peritoneal cells (1 h at 37 °C)

Concentration (μg/ml)	CHSA* (0% acylated)	LCHSA** (22% acylated)	LCHSA (82% acylated)
1	3.26 ± 0.25***	6.94 ± 0.58***	23.44 ± 1.05***
10	0.65	3.65	10.44
100	0.23	1.83	5.31

The results are expressed as percentage of protein attached
  *CHSA = human serum exposed to solvent mixtures
 **LCHSA = lauroylated HSA
***Number of experiments = 5

lymphatic through the thoracic duct and from there to the systemic circulation. Unfortunately data concerning transport in the portal vein cannot be entirely reliable, since antigen will recirculate from the systemic circulation through the mesenteric arterial supply. Consequently we investigated the transport of antigen in the mesenteric lymph, by cannulation of the intestinal lymph trunk, before its entry into the thoracic duct. The lymph was collected after injection into the bowel of radio iodinated protein antigens. The lymph recovered during the period 2½-3 h after injection of the antigens was fractioned over a Sephadex G-25 column and the proportion of counts in the protein peaks compared. After the injection of radio iodinated HSA into the bowel a small proportion ($2.77 \pm 0.69\%$ n = 5) of the total radioactivity lay in the protein peak of the lymph. However when LCHSA was injected, a significantly lower percentage of total radioactivity ($0.375 \pm 0.27\%$ n = 4, p $\prec 0.001$) was found in the protein peak of the lymph. The reduction in the lymphatic transport of acylated protein is perhaps surprising since lipoproteins are transported in the intestinal lymph, as is also a proportion of the free absorbed fatty acid. However, this reduction in the amount of absorbed undigested immunogen in the lymph could be explained by fewer molecules penetrating the mucosa because of the tendency of the molecules to aggregate, and also by the greater tendency of any molecules successfully penetrating the mucosa to attach to cell surfaces because of their hydrophobic fatty acid side-chains.

Anticomplementary activity

We have also investigated the anticomplementary activity of LCHSA by a modified Mayer technique. We found that all acylated proteins tested showed some anticomplementary activity. The effect increased with the degree of acylation (Table 2). The intrinsic anticomplementary activity of the conjugated antigens and the enhanced antibody response which they induce may be compared to the action of endotoxin as an extrinsic immunological adjuvant since the anticomplementary activity of endotoxin is related to its fatty acid side-chains (Gewurz et al., 1968). The manner of reactivity with complement is being examined further but if it represents an activation of the alternate pathway comparable to that produced by endotoxin, the immunogen would itself provide the two signals postulated as necessary for B-cell activation, namely, an antigenic signal and a signal from the C3 component of complement (Dukor and

Table 2 Complement activity (CH 50) of guinea pig serum after explosure to lipid conjugated HSA*

	CHSA	LCHSA	LCHSA	LCHSA	CFD
Percentage acylation	0	36	60	82	—
Residual CHSO units	12.5	9.7	8.5	3.4	12.5

*All protein solutions were at a concentration of 5 mg/ml in complement fixing diluent (CFD), reacting with five times the volume of complement diluted 1:10

Hartmann, 1973). Such a characteristic would further help to explain the greater immunological effectiveness of the smaller percentage of acylated molecules absorbed from the gut.

Intrinsic adjuvanticity and immunogenicity

These experiments demonstrate that it is possible to induce high levels of antibody by introducing lipid-conjugated protein into the bowel. The increased immunogenicity is consistent with the adjuvant effects of extrinsic lipid and lipidophilic substances on antibody production but is here related to integral molecular features of intrinsic adjuvanticity (Dresser, 1962). The reduction in the enhanced antibody formation with increased acylation is probably due to obscuring of important determinants by the attached fatty acid side-chains. Coon and Hunter who were able to establish delayed-type hypersensitivity in guinea pigs with acylated bovine serum albumin did not induce detectable antibody with the very highly acylated proteins they found necessary for this effect.

The increased immunogenicity of acylated protein is thus associated with increased molecular aggregation and cellular adherence, and an anticomplementary effect, but decreased transport in the protein peak of fractionated lymph.

SITES OF ANTIBODY SYNTHESIS

In defining the possible sites of antibody production after antigenic stimulation in the gut, we must consider the immune apparatus associated with the intestine and the distribution of antigen molecules. Antigen may become directly associated with immunologically competent cells (ICC) in the bowel wall or may be drained by lymphatics or tributaries of the portal vein. Antigen in the lymphatics may come in contact with ICC in the mesenteric lymph nodes but the anatomy of the lymphatics is such that many molecules will bypass the nodes and will be carried directly into the intestinal trunk, thus reaching the thoracic duct and systemic circulation without having passed through lymphoid tissue. Alternatively antigen in the portal venous system will be filtered in the liver and a proportion will reach the systemic circulation. Antigen reaching the systemic circulation by either route may reach other antibody forming tissue, principally the spleen, on recirculation.

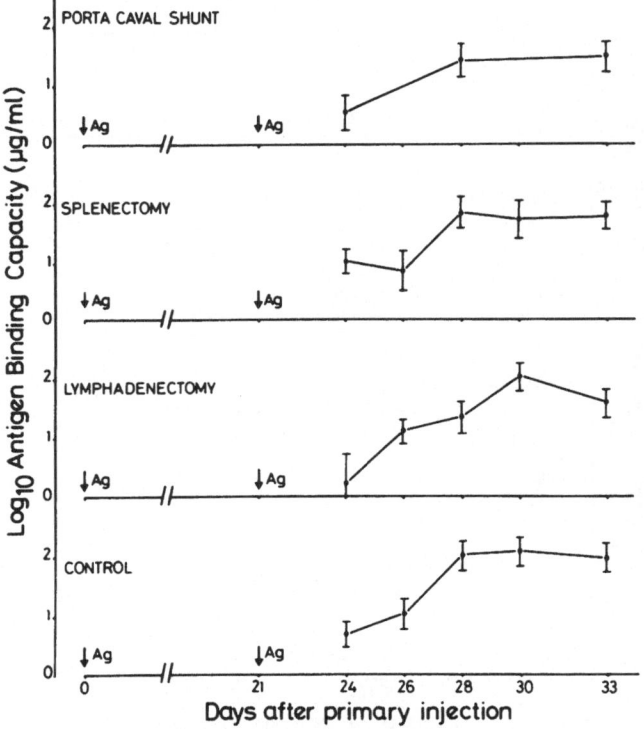

Figure 5 Rat secondary antibody responses to intrabowel lauroylated HSA (10 mg + 1 mg) after portacaval shunt, splenectomy, lymphadenectomy or sham operation.

Antibody formation after removal of lymphoid tissue or altered portal circulation

In an attempt to define the site of antibody synthesis in the gut associated immune tissues we have performed a series of experiments to remove the effect of separate parts of this immune apparatus systematically. These experiments were performed after (i) splenectomy, or (ii) excision of the mesenteric lymph nodes with careful preservation of the intestinal lymph trunk, or (iii) bypass of the liver by means of a portacaval shunt procedure. The mesenteric lymph nodes were removed by careful dissection of the peritoneum covering the nodes, followed by excision of the nodes. Portacaval shunt was performed by ligation of the portal vein in the porta hepatis and transection of the vein. The proximal end of the vein is then anastomosed end-to-side to the inferior vena cava. There

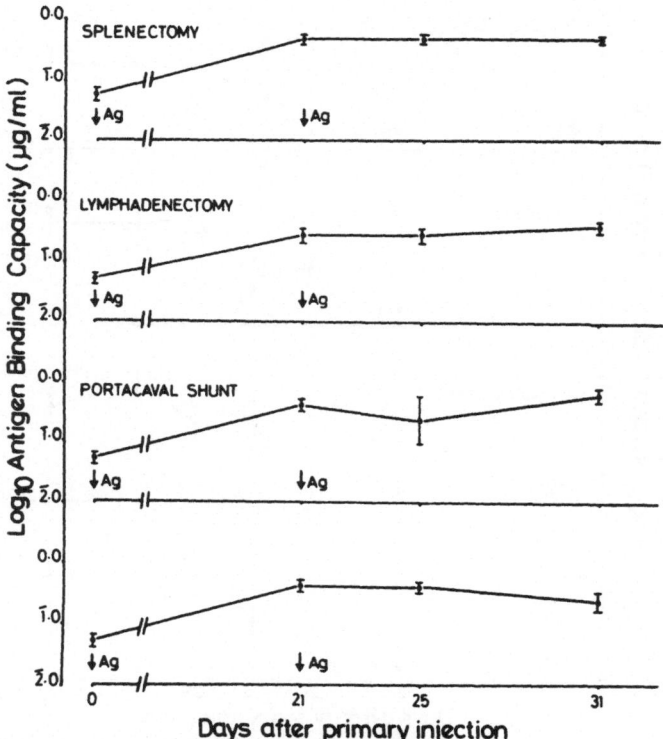

Figure 6 Rat primary and secondary antibody responses to intrabowel diphtheria toxoid (400 μg and 100 μg) after splenectomy, lymphadenectomy, portacaval shunt or sham operation.

130

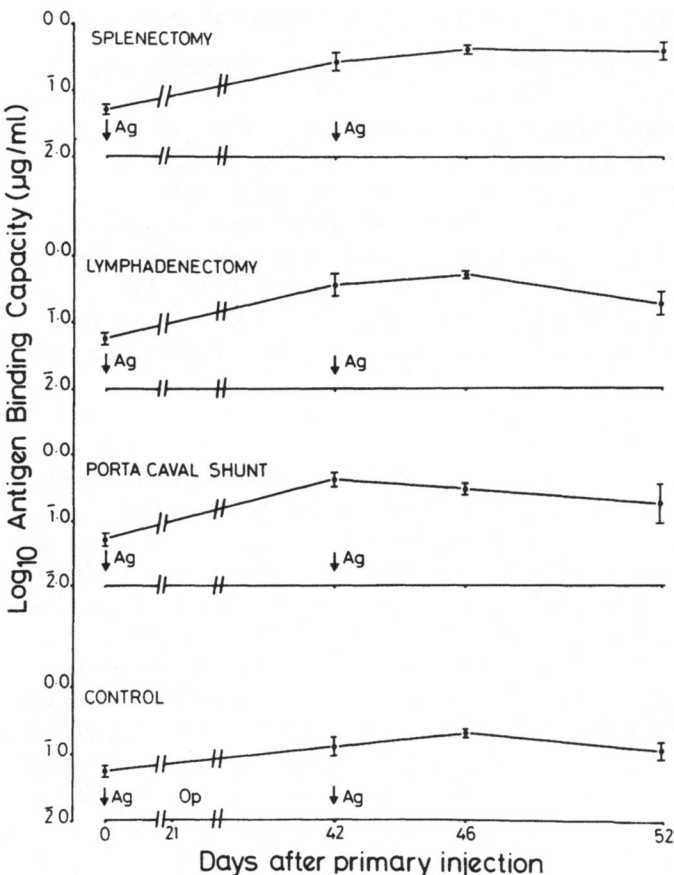

Figure 7 Rat primary and secondary antibody responses to intrabowel diphtheria toxoid (400 µg or 100 µg). Primary stimulation was 21 days before and secondary stimulation 21 days after operation.

were two series of experiments, one in which the operation was performed after sensitization with antigen, and the other in which the operation was performed before initial sensitization with antigen. Two antigens were investigated, diphtheria toxoid and lipid conjugated HSA. The results of these experiments demonstrate that none of these procedures influenced the development of primary or secondary antibody responses to these antigens (Figures 5-7).

Localization of antibody by the fluorescent antibody technique

Finally, after immunization with diphtheria toxoid into the bowel lumen, organs were excised from the animals and subjected to immunofluorescent examination by the sandwich technique with fluorescein-labelled diphtheria antitoxin to detect cell associated antibody.

Sections of liver, spleen, mesenteric lymph nodes and small and large bowel wall were examined. This study demonstrated that there were many fluorescent cells in the subcapsular areas of the mesenteric lymph nodes (in a typical 'string of pearls' distribution); and also in the lamina propria of the small bowel. There were very few fluorescent cells in the large bowel wall, Peyer's patches and spleen, and none at all in the liver.

CONCLUSION

We would conclude from our work that antigen is absorbed from the bowel lumen. It is likely that immunogenic molecules penetrate the intestinal mucosa to reach the lamina propria of the small gut wall.

Although our work is incomplete at present our results suggest that immunogenic molecules then travel by the intestinal lymphatics to the regional lymph nodes. Macrophages with cytophilic antibody on their surface or antibody forming cells themselves can subsequently be found in the nodes. Antibody is thus probably synthesized both in the lamina propria of the small intestine and in the mesenteric lymph nodes. With the antigens that we have used we have no evidence to suggest that either the spleen, colon or the liver play an essential role in antibody synthesis following antigenic stimulation in the gastrointestinal tract.

ACKNOWLEDGEMENTS

We are indebted to the Editor of 'Immunology', for permission to reproduce the data in Figures 3 and 4 and Tables 1 and 2, and also Dr Valentine French, Dept. of Experimental Pathology, University of Birmingham for a gift of fluorescein labelled diphtheria antitoxin.

References

Coon, J. and Hunter, R. (1973). Selective induction of delayed hypersensitivity by a lipid-conjugated protein antigen which is localized in thymus-dependent lymphoid tissue. J. Immunol., **110**, 183

Dresser, D. W. (1962). Specific inhibition of antibody production. II

Paralysis induced in adult mice by small quantities of protein antigen. Immunology, **5**, 378

Dukor, P. and Hartmann, K. U. (1973). Hypothesis. bound C3 as the second signal for B-cell activation. Cell. Immunol., **7**, 349

Frei, P. C. (1964). Influence de la dimension des particles d'un antigene proteinique sur la response ou la tolerance immunitaires. C.R. Soc. Suisse Physiol., **64**, 124

Gewurz, H., Mergenhagen, S. E., Nowotny, A. and Phillips, J. R. (1968). Interactions of the complement system with native and chemically modified endotoxins. J. Bact., **95**, 397

Heatley, R. V. and Stark, J. M. (1975). Immunogenicity of lipid-conjugated protein in the intestine. Immunology, **29**, 143

Mitchison, N. A. (1971). The carrier effect in the secondary response to hapten-protein conjugates. I The measurement of the effect with transferred cells and objections to the local environment hypothesis. Eur. J. Immunol., **1**, 10

Spitznagel, J. K. and Allison, A. C. (1970). Mode of action of adjuvants. Effects on antibody response to macrophage- associated bovine serum albumin. J. Immunol., **104**, 128

13

Natural antibodies and the intestinal flora in rodents

A. LEE and M. C. FOO

For the past 6 years a research team headed by Professor G. N. Cooper has studied the immunology and microbiology of the gastrointestinal tract. The immune response of animals following injection of antigen into the small intestine had earlier been investigated by Robertson and Cooper 1972, 1973; Cooper et al., 1967; Cooper and Thonard, 1967 who demonstrated that following antigenic stimulation via the intestinal epithelium, the splenic response contributed most to the circulating antibody responses of rats. However, with a technique enumerating rosette-forming cells in dispersed suspensions of lymphoid cells from mesenteric lymph nodes, intestinal lamina propria and submucosal tissues, these workers detected significant increases in the level of cells synthesizing the three major classes of immunoglobulins in local and peripheral lymphoid tissue.

In general terms the primary response of mesenteric lymph nodes following intestinal antigenic stimulation was similar to that observed in the spleen or other lymph nodes when antigen is given parenterally, showing the characteristic change from IgM to IgG antibody formation. In the intestinal submucosa and lamina propria IgA-rosette-forming cells were most numerous but a significant IgG response also occurred. IgA-rosette-forming cells also appeared in the spleen following immunization via the intestinal route. It was concluded that cells of the lamina propria do not contribute substantially to serum IgA antibody levels. The spleen and mesenteric lymph nodes appeared to constitute the major sources of circulating IgA antibody. It was questioned whether oral immunization offered any major advantage over parenteral routes in terms of inducing IgA antibody formation at the mucosal surface.

The contributions of the authors to this research programme have been confined to investigation of the microbiology of the intestine. However

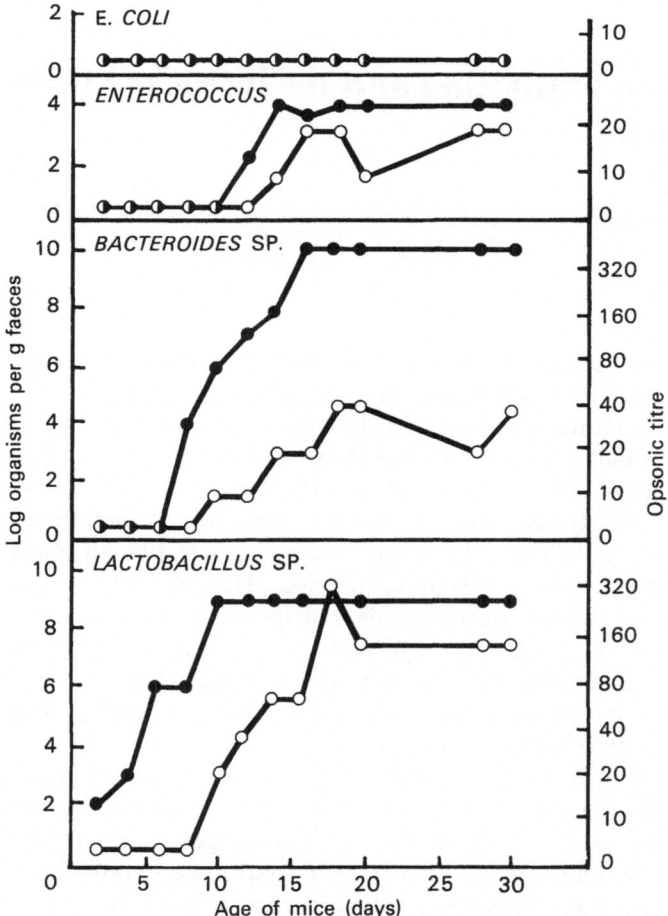

Figure 1 Colonization of intestinal organisms and development of homologous serum opsonizing antibody in newborn SPF mice. viable organisms •, serum opsonins o. Each point represents the mean of figures obtained from 10 litters of mice.

136

some results on the appearance of natural antibodies against intestinal bacteria may be of interest to workers in the field of antigen absorption by the gut.

The bowel is continually bombarded with antigenic stimuli; one main source of antigens is the food, the other is the normal resident microflora. It is not always appreciated that the intestinal content from the terminal ileum downward is almost entirely made up of viable bacteria. Some absorption of antigens from these organisms necessarily occurs and one end result is the presence of natural antibody in the serum. These 'natural antibodies' are immunoglobulins found in relatively low and constant levels in individuals of the same species living in a particular environment (Boyden, 1966). They may be specific for a particular microbial species or may cross-react with antigens of other, non-commensal organisms (Kunin et al., 1962) or even host tissue components such as the blood group substances and Forssman antigens (Springer et al., 1959).

The appearance of natural antibody against intestinal organisms has been found to follow the colonization of the neonatal intestine with bacteria (Foo et al., 1974). Microorganisms appear in the intestines of young animals in a constant sequence. This is illustrated in Figure 1. Mice were exsanguinated at different times after birth and the pooled sera from single litters were tested for opsonizing antibody activity. The number of microorganisms in the intestinal contents of these same animals was determined by viable counts on various selective media. The organisms appeared in the gastrointestinal tract at specific times after birth and rapidly increased in numbers to normal adult levels. Specific serum opsonins in mice did not develop until several days after the organism had established in the intestine, but they reached normal levels at about the 20th day of life; i.e. around weaning time. Note the high level of antibody against Lactobacilli, the first organism to colonize. This will be referred to below.

Experiments were also carried out to determine the effect of delaying the colonization of the intestinal tract. The results of one of these experiments are shown in Figure 2. Twenty male and eighty female mice were housed in different cages and given penicillin in their drinking water for 4 weeks, the period necessary to completely eliminate Lactobacillus from the intestines. Four randomly selected female mice were exsanguinated to confirm that the sera did not contain opsonins for the organism, thus obviating the possibility of transfer of maternal antibody. At this stage the mice were mated, housed in individual cages and

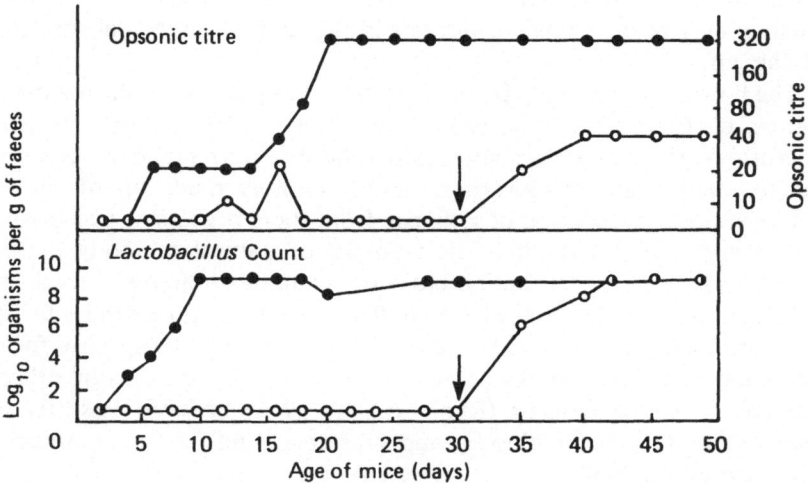

Figure 2 Colonization of intestines with Lactobacilli and development of homologous serum opsonizing antibody in newborn mice.•, normal baby mice; o, baby mice born with Lactobacilli in their gastrointestinal tract and maintained on penicillin treatment. At day 30 (arrow) penicillin treatment was withheld from remaining litters.

maintained on penicillin. Following birth individual litters were killed at various times and the levels of antibodies and concentration of bacteria were measured. From Figure 2 the following observations may be made

(i)   The pencillin treatment effectively prevented colonization of the intestines with Lactobacilli whereas these organisms reached high levels (ca. 10_9 organisms /g of intestinal homogenates) by the tenth day of life of normal mice.

(ii)   Animals in which colonization was prevented did not develop serum opsonins for Lactobacilli but once these organisms became established (after day 30) opsonins appeared and reached constant titres within 10 days.

(iii) In normal animals, wherein Lactobacilli reached high levels within 10 days of birth, the serum opsonin titres were significantly higher than in those animals which were colonized by the organisms after 30 days of life. Consistently it appeared as though early colonization of the intestine resulted in higher titres of natural antibody in adult life. In those mice treated with pencillin from birth Escherichia coli established in the large bowel in high numbers much earlier than in normal animals, consequently the level of natural antibody was found to be increased.

138

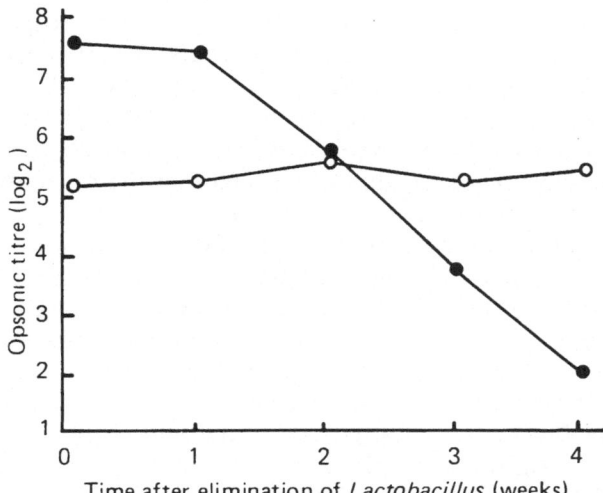

Figure 3 Serum opsonin titres of mice given penicillin to eliminate Lactobacillus sp. from the intestinal tract. •, Lactobacillus opsonins; ō, E.coli. opsonins. A minimum of 10 mice were tested at each time.

The next question asked was whether constant antigen absorption was needed to maintain these levels of natural antibody. Figure 3 shows results of one of a series of experiments in which the normal flora was altered by antibiotic treatment. Mice were housed in sterile cages with sterile food and bedding, and drinking water containing penicillin. The cages, plus bedding, food and drinking water, were changed every alternate day while faeces were collected aseptically from each mouse daily to culture for Lactobacilli and E. col. Mice were exsanguinated at different times after it had been confirmed that the organism in question had been eliminated from the intestine. The sera were then tested individually for opsonic activity against both bacterial species. As is seen in Figure 3 serum opsonins for Lactobacillus began to decline about 2 weeks after its elimination from the gastrointestinal tract and by the end of 4 weeks they were below the limit of detection in 6 of the 10 animals tested. However the sera of these animals retained E. coli opsonins at the same level throughout the period of examination. Similar results were found in experiments with kanamycin which eliminated E. coli but not the Lactobacilli; only the E. coli opsonin level decreased. Thus it appears as though antigen has to be constantly present in the intestine to maintain levels of natural antibody.

139

This need for continuous antigen absorption was also seen in a different series of experiments. Mice were fed suspensions of Hyphomicrobium sp., an unusual microorganism first isolated from a hydroelectric pipe in Tasmania (Tyler and Marchall 1967). Not surprisingly, the normal mouse has not detectable antibody to this organism. The animals were given 1×10^7 organisms by stomach tube daily for 15 days. Faecal cultures indicated that the organism survived for only a few hours after each inoculation. At least 5 mice were randomly selected at various times during and after this period and their sera tested for Hyphomicrobium opsonins. Fifty days later the remaining mice were again fed daily for 15 days with living suspensions and the sera from randomly selected animals were again measured for opsonic activity against Hyphomicrobium sp. over a period of 50 days. The results are summarized in Figure 4. Opsonizing antibody appeared within 4 days of the first dose of the organisms and reached a peak at day 14. As soon as the organisms were withheld the antibody level declined below the level of detection within 3 weeks. When the oral dose was given over the second 15-day period, development and appearance of Hyphomicrobium followed a similar course.

It is relevant to studies into oral immunisation to ask why is the

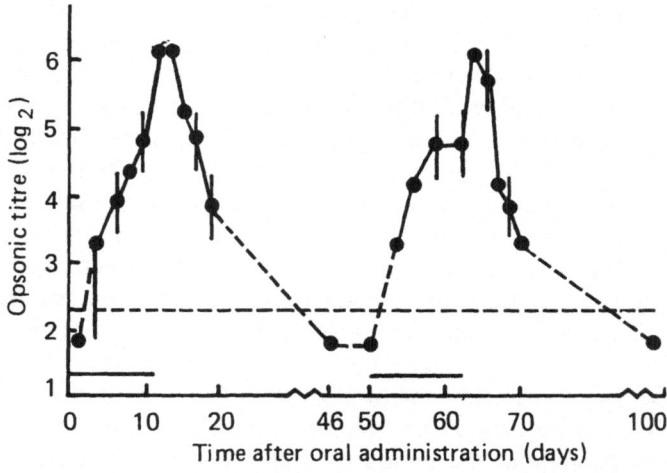

Figure 4 Homologous serum opsonins in adult mice following continuous oral feeding of living Hyphomicrobium sp. The horizontal bars indicate the periods of oral feeding and the broken line is the limit of detectability of the opsonins. A minimum of five mice were tested at each time.

140

response to these 'natural antigens' in the intestine so poor? As is seen above, only low levels of immunoglobulin are induced and there is no evidence for the development of immunological memory. Presumably this relates to the amount of antigen absorbed by the intestine. Results of experiments of other workers in which antigen has been artifically introduced into the intestinal tract have shown characteristic primary and secondary responses and high levels of antibody. Cooper et al. (1967) injected Salmonella organisms into isolated loops of small intestine and demonstrated a good immune response. In this case the antigen was trapped and so larger amounts were presumably available for absorption by the gut. In the normal animal the passage of material through the small intestine is so rapid that it limits opportunity of absorption. The good immune response to intraintestinal injection of sheep red blood cells reported by Robertson and Cooper (1972) was possibly due to the high concentration of absorbable antigen; the cells presumably lyse in the intestinal lumen. Also the trauma of a laparotomy possibly resulted in a slowing of intestinal mobility and hence prolonged opportunity for antigen absorption.

Large amounts of bacteria are present in the bowel and so it is worth considering why so little antigen is apparently absorbed. As has been mentioned any antigen introduced into the small bowel has very little opportunity of passing the mucosa because of rapid transit time. The majority of the indigenous microflora exist in the caecum and colon where the epithelial surfaces are continuous and overlaid by large amounts of mucin which would hinder absorption. Also the mucosal surfaces of these areas have a very specific dense microflora which may prevent other organisms from coming in contact with the mucosa.

The experiments of Tlaskalova et al. (1970) are pertinent to these discussions. These workers monocontaminated germ-free piglets orally with indigenous E. coli and obtained a good immune response. The author has observed that in similarly monocontaminated germ-free mice and rats, the E. coli colonizes the whole of the intestinal tract. Thus in the piglets it is likely that there was continual presence of antigen in the small bowel and no competition from mucosal organisms, hence the heightened immune response.

A paper by Triger et al. (1972) suggests that the liver may be influencing the level of antibodies to the antigens present in the intestine. It was shown that during the breakdown of liver function, antibody levels to members of the gastrointestinal flora increase significantly. The authors suggest that antigen which enters the intestinal tissue is not taken

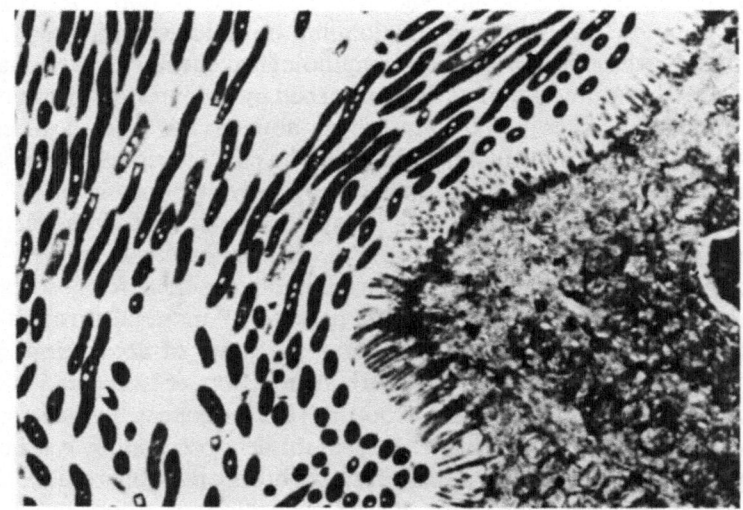

Figure 5 Cross section of normal rat caecum through crypt; magnification: × 8000.

up by macrophages in situ but enters the portal circulation and is rapidly removed by the liver.

For the reasons discussed above it is apparent that only minute amounts of antigen are available to bind with and subsequently stimulate lymphoid cells in the intestinal tissue. While this is sufficient to evoke an initial response by these cells it may not cause proliferation or differentiation which are considered essential for normal antibody formation and immunological memory.

In conclusion it is important to remind workers interested in experimental antigenic absorption across the intestinal mucosa of the presence of dense populations of bacteria associated with the mucosa in animals commonly used for these experiments. Certainly, the majority of these organisms are in the large bowel and so their influence on antigen uptake is doubtful; however there are large numbers of bacteria found in the terminal ileum of normal rodents. The presence of a mucosal associated flora has only recently been demonstrated (Davis et al., 1972; Leach et al., 1973). The intestine contains a variety of individual ecological niches which often favour the growth of only one type of bacterium. This is illustrated in Figure 5. Thus the intestine of the rat can be divided into six distinct areas with regard to bacteria on the mucosa. The upper small bowel is clear of organisms but the five other regions have characteristic populations of different bacterial species (Lee and Leach, unpublished observations).

This paper has looked at the consequences of the normal antigen presence in the gastrointestinal tract. Hopefully it may have raised some questions which will prove valuable for those concerned with the study of antigen absorption by the gut.

References

Boyden, S. V. (1966). Natural antibodies and the immune response. Adv. Immunol., **5**, 1

Cooper, G. N., Halliday, W. J. and Thonard, J. C. (1967). Immunological reactivity associated with antigens in the intestinal tract of rats. J. Path. Bact., **93**, 223

Cooper, G. N. and Thonard, J. C. (1967). Serum antibody responses to intestinal implantation of antigens in rats. J. Path. Bact., **93**, 213

Davis, C. P., Mulcahy, D., Takeuchi, A. and Savage, D. C. (1972). Location and description of spiral-shaped microorganisms in the normal rat caecum. Infect. Immun. **6**, 184

Foo, M. C., Lee, A. and Cooper, G. N. (1974). Natural antibodies and the intestinal flora of rodents. Aust. J. Exp. Biol. Sci., **52**, 321

Kunin, C. M., Beard, M. V. and Malmagyi, H. E. (1962). Evidence for a common hapten associated with enterotoxin fraction of E. coli and other Enterobacteriaceae. Proc. Soc. Exp. Biol. Med., **111**, 160

Leach, W. D., Lee. A. and Stubbs, R. P. (1973). Localization of bacteria in the gastrointestinal tract: a possible explanation of intestinal spirochaetosis. Infect. Immun., **7**, 961

Robertson, P. W. and Cooper, G. N. (1972). Immune responses in intestinal tissues to particulate antigens. Plaque-forming and rosette-forming responses in rats. Aust. J. Exp. Biol. Med. Sci., **50**, 703

Robertson, P. W. and Cooper, G. N. (1973). Immune responses in intestinal tissues to particulate antigens. Development of cells forming different classes of antibody in primary and secondary responses. Aust. J. Exp. Biol. Med. Sci., **51**, 575

Springer, G. F., Honton, R. E. and Forbes, M. (1959). Origin of anti-human blood group B agglutinins in germ-free chicks. Ann. N.Y. Acad. Sci., **78**, 272

Tlaskalova, H., Kamarytova, V., Mandel L. et al. (1972). Folio Biologica, **xvi**, 177

Triger, D. R., Alp, M. H. and Wright, R. (1972). Bacterial and dietary antibodies in liver disease. Lancet, i, 60

Tyler, P. A. and Marshall, K. C. (1967). Pheomorphy in stalked, budding bacteria. J. Bact., 93, 1132

14

Delayed-hypersensitivity reactions in the small intestine

ANNE FERGUSON

INTRODUCTION

Lymphoid cells of the small intestine are present both as aggregates, the Peyer's patches, and as single cells dispersed among the absorptive and stromal tissues of the mucosa. In the lamina propria there are lymphocytes, plasma cells, macrophages, eosinophils and mast cells and many medium-sized lymphocytes are present between the enterocytes — intraepithelial (IE) lymphocytes. The presence of thymus dependent (T) and thymus independent (B) lymphocytes in the intestine, has been demonstrated by morphological examination of the tissues of thymus deprived rodents (Ferguson and Parrott, 1972a), and by studies of cell traffic to the intestine using radioisotope labelling and immunofluoresence (Parrott and Ferguson, 1974; Guy-Grande et al., 1974). the Peyer's patches are populated by small T and B lymphocytes (as are other peripheral lymphoid tissues such as lymph nodes). However, the lymphocytes and plasma cells of the villi are derived from large lymphocytes — immunoblasts — probably both T and B. The thymus dependence of some intestinal IE lymphocytes has recently been demonstrated by the findings of low IE lymphocyte counts in thymus deprived mice (Ferguson and Parrott, 1972a), and by the homing of radioisotope labelled T immunoblasts to the intraepithelial site (Guy-Grande et al., 1974).

Since the intestinal mucosa contains T cells, it may be the site of protective cell mediated immune (CMI) reactions, or of disease due to local delayed hypersensitivity. This paper describes how CMI reactions may influence structure and functions of the non-lymphoid components of the small intestine, and illustrates the clinical applications of this experimental work in relation to the intestinal lesion of coeliac disease.

INTESTINAL ALLOGRAFT REJECTION — A MODEL OF LOCAL DELAYED HYPERSENSITIVITY

The small intestine is the target of an immune reaction in graft-versus-host disease and a similar mechanism causes rejection of an intestinal allograft. We have studied rejection of mouse small intestine by using heterotopically transplanted grafts of fetal intestine (Ferguson and Parrott, 1972b; Ferguson and Parrott, 1973), and have found this

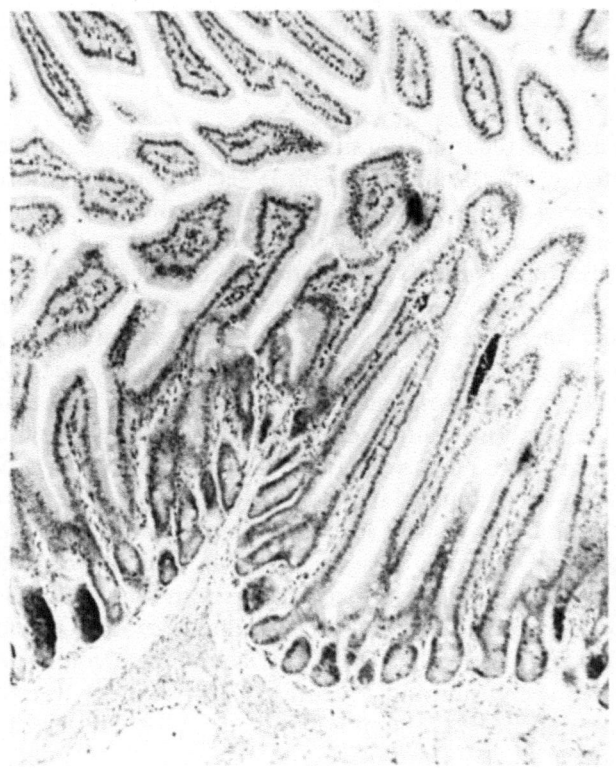

Figure 1 Isograft of mouse small intestine

model to have several advantages. The operative technique is simple and inexpensive; the transplanted tissue is sterile and has never contained food, so that any pathological features can be attributed directly to rejection; the results of experiments with thymus deprived animals indicate that the reaction is thymus-dependent (Ferguson and Parrott, 1973); and since mucosal destruction precedes the appearance of anti-graft antibodies in the serum (Elves and Ferguson, 1976), we have confirmed that the reaction is mediated by lymphocytes.

Methods

Animals used for these experiments were mice of the strain CBA, Balb-c and C3H-Bi, maintained in the Department of Bacteriology and Immunology, University of Glasgow. The technique for grafting fetal intestin has been described in detail elsewhere. (Ferguson and Parrott, 1972b; Ferguson, 1973). Pregnant mice were killed on the 18th or 19th day of gestation; the fetal small intestine was dissected out and cut into segments 5-10 mm in length; and pieces of small intestine were implanted under the kidney capsules of adult recipient mice (two grafts per mouse). Groups of recipient mice were killed at intervals after graft implantation and the grafts, with a little kidney tissue, were dissected out, fixed in formol saline, routinely embedded and sectioned at three

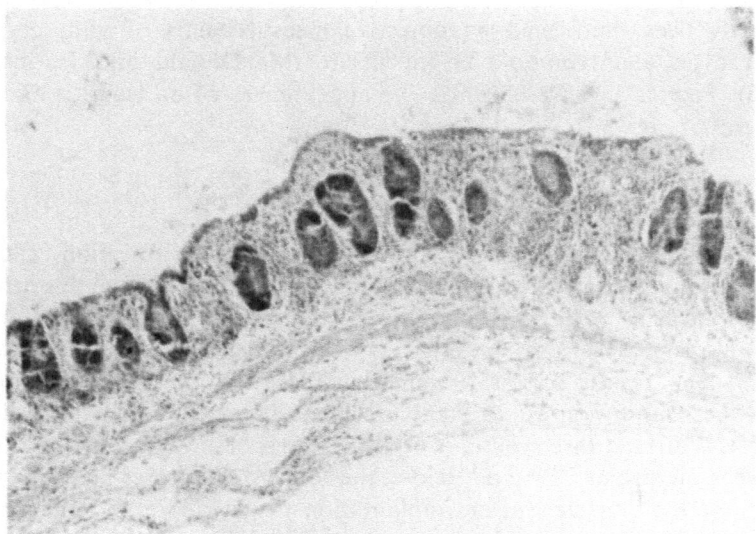

Figure 2 Rejection of an allograft of mouse small intestine — grade 'flat'

levels. Adequate histological preparations were obtained in around 90% of experiments and the results described below are based on the findings in 224 allografts, 58 isografts and 29 specimens of normal small intestine.

Histopathology of rejection

The sequence of events which leads to rejection has been identical in all the strain combinations studied, although the time course is influenced by histocompatibility differences between donor and host strains. Five morphological grades have been described (Ferguson and Parrott, 1973).

Normal for age, with villi normal, crypts short and virtually no plasma cells or lymphocytes in the lamina propria.

L+, lymphocyte infiltration of the lamina propria with many lymphocytes and pyroninophilic blast cells in lymphatics.

L+ +, dense lymphocyte infiltration throughout the full thickness of the graft, but villi still recognizable.

Flat, villi very short or absent, although epithelium and crypts are still present — subtotal villous atrophy.

Submucosa, epithelium and lamina propria destroyed so that the graft consists of smooth muscle heavily infiltrated with lymphocytes and plasma cells.

These subjective impressions of the changes in villi and crypts have recently been confirmed by objective measurements of villi, crypts, enterocytes and lymphoid cell infiltrate (MacDonald and Ferguson, 1976). Figures 1 and 2 illustrate the appearances of an isograft and an allograft.

The effects of rejection on single crypts

From standard light microscopy it seems that rejection causes lengthening of the crypts of Lieberkuhn. We have investigated this aspect further by using colchicine to produce metaphase arrest, and by counting the numbers of mitoses in single crypts. (MacDonald and Ferguson, 1977). The results so far obtained indicate that in neonatal mouse intestine, and in isografts of fetal intestine, the rate of entry of cells into mitosis is around three cells per crypt per hour. However, in allografts, between the strains CBA and Balb-c, the value is 13 mitoses per crypt per hour on the 5th day after implantation — evidence of true crypt hyperplasia with 5 times the normal cell production rate.

Summary of the effects of rejection on the mucosa

This thymus dependent, cell-mediated immune reaction against small intestinal antigens produces lymphocyte infiltration of the lamina propria with crypt hyperplasia and, later, ulceration; usually these are accompanied by villous atrophy and high intraepithelial lymphocyte counts but rejection does not affect the appearance of individual enterocytes, and plasma cells are present only at the late, submucosa stage. Similar findings have been reported for rejection of small intestine in other species and in graft-versus-host disease (in which the small intestinal lesion produces a malabsorption syndrome) (Hedberg et al., 1968).

It has not yet been established how the CMI reaction produces changes in the architecture and functions of the small intestine. By analogy with CMI in other tissues, the effector mechanisms may be either cytotoxic T cells or lymphokines (factors secreted by activated T cells on contact with specific antigen). If lymphokines are involved, then the harmful CMI response need not necessarily be directed against the intestinal tissues per se. Similar lymphokine secretion would occur when T cells interact with other intestinal antigens in the mucosa (e.g. parasites, foods).

THYMUS DEPENDENCE OF PARTIAL VILLOUS ATROPHY IN A PARASITE INFECTION

Partial or subtotal villous atrophy with crypt hyperplasia is common to many clinical and experimental conditions including helminth parasite infection. It has usually been assumed that the intestinal lesion is produced by toxins from the worms, but it is equally possible that a local hypersensitivity reaction contributes to the pathology. We infected several groups of rats with the parasite Nippostrongylus brasiliensis, and confirmed that this infection produced partial villous atrophy in affected areas of the small intestine of normal rats (Figure 3). However, when the infected rats had previously been depleted of T cells by thymectomy and irradiation, the expected enteropathy was absent in 70% of experimental animals (Figure 4) (Ferguson and Jarrett, 1975). This local 'enteropathic' immune response could be mediated by thymus dependent antibodies, T lymphocytes, or other cell type such as mast cells. We found that passive immunization with hyperimmune anti-nippostrongylus serum did not restore the capacity of worm infection to damage the small bowel in thymus-deprived rats (Ferguson and Jarrett, 1975), and this provides

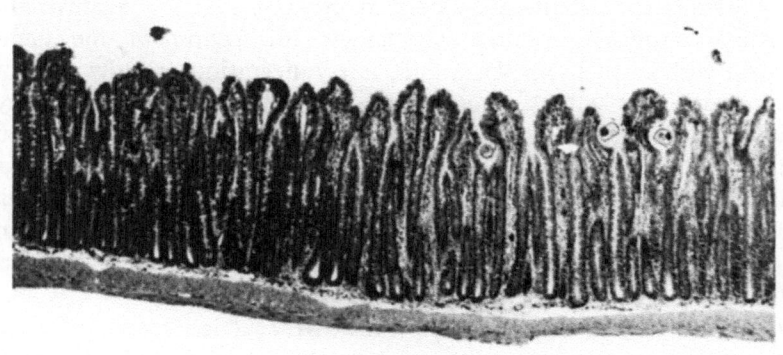

Figure 3 Partial villous atrophy in the small intestine of a rat on the 10th day after infection with 4000 Nippostrongylus brasiliensis larvae

limited evidence implicating lymphocyte related factors rather than antibodies as the cause of the intestinal lesion in immunologically intact animals.

IS THERE DELAYED HYPERSENSITIVITY TO GLUTEN IN COELIAC DISEASE?

Coeliac disease is a permanent condition in which the patient usually presents with malabsorption, but may be asymptomatic; a biopsy of the proximal small intestine is flat with no villi, long crypts and intense lymphoid cell infiltrate; and there is clinical, biochemical and morphological improvement when gluten (wheat, rye, oats and barley) is withdrawn from the diet. The nature of the gluten intolerance is still disputed but there is increasing evidence in favour of an immunological basis to the disease (Hekkens and Pena, 1974; Ferguson, 1976). In untreated coeliac disease, patients may have very high levels of serum IgA and the lamina propria is packed with plasma cells, the increase affecting cells of the IgA, IgM and IgG classes. These patients have abnormally high titres of antibody to gluten or gliadin in serum and in the intestinal secretions (Ferguson and Carswell, 1972), but they also

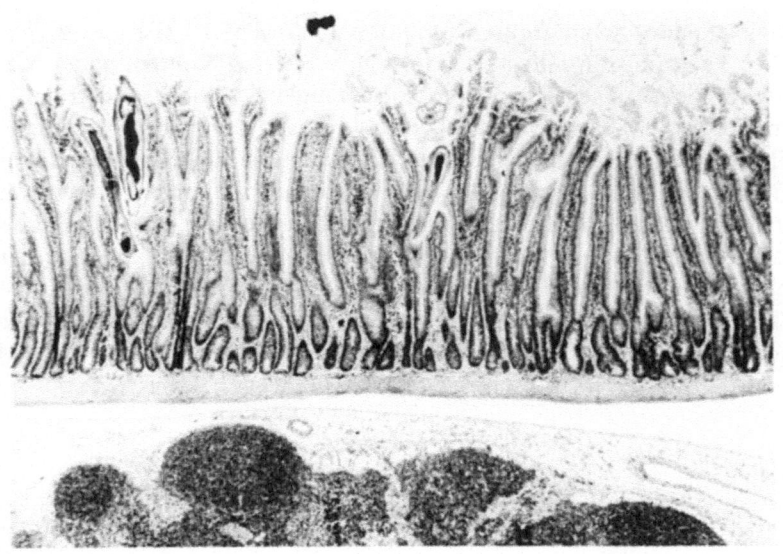

Figure 4 Completely normal morphology of the small intestine on the 19th day after infection of a thymus deprived rat with 4000 Nippostrongylus brasiliensis larvae

have similar antibodies to other foods such as cows' milk and egg, foods which they tolerate normally.

Changes in the number and distribution of intestinal lymphocytes are also present in coeliac disease. Lamina propria lymphocytes are reduced in number (Holmes et al., 1973) and intraepithelial (IE) lymphocyte counts are increased (Ferguson and Murray, 1971). IE lymphocyte counts fall after gluten withdrawal (Ferguson and Murray, 1971) and (in adults) rise within 24 hours of an oral gluten challenge (Ferguson, 1974). Several workers have looked for evidence of CMI to gluten. Intradermal skin tests with gluten were negative (Asquith, 1974) and culture of peripheral blood lymphocytes with gluten or gliadin has given completely negative results in some hands, although one group have reported gluten-related blast transformation in 16% of untreated coeliac patients (Asquith, 1974).

We recently extended the investigation of CMI to gluten in coeliac disease by studying the functions of lymphocytes within the small intestinal mucosa. Fragments of intestine (with their contained lymphocytes) were cultured in the presence and absence of alpha-gliadin, and subsequently the culture medium was assayed for a lymphokine-like activity (leukocyte migration inhibition factor, MIF) (Ferguson et al., 1976). The results are illustrated in Figure 5. Of 29 control patients and 15 with coeliac disease in whom culture media without added antigen were studied, MIF activity was detected in only one control patient (a child with unexplained diarrhoea). Culture with alpha-gliadin did not influence the subsequent leukocyte migration in six control patients and in two gluten-free diet treated coeliac patients. However, in five of the six untreated coeliac patients, 5 h culture of jejunal mucosa with alpha-gliadin produced 30% or more migration inhibition.

These preliminary results accord with the concept that, in coeliac disease, the fully documented humoral immune reactions may be

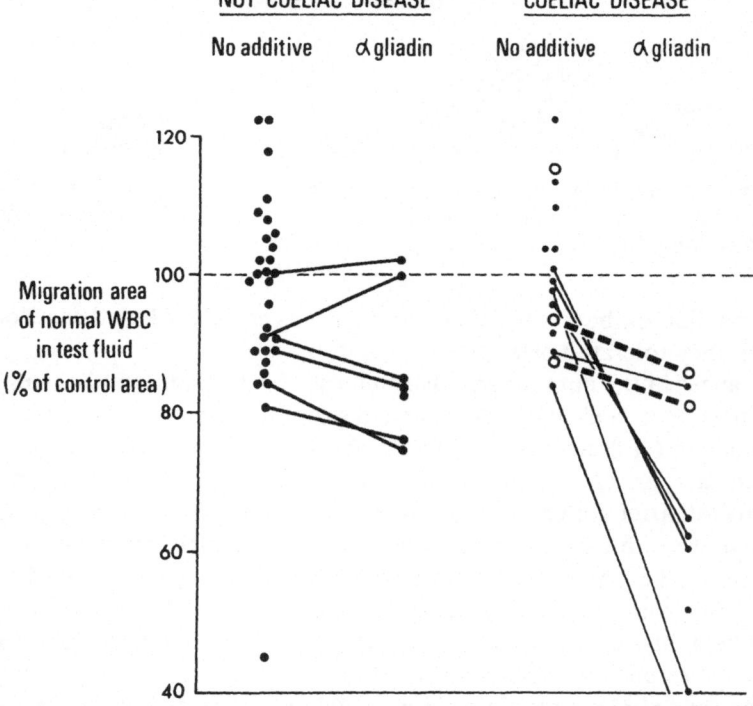

Figure 5 Migration of normal human white blood cells in test culture medium, expressed as percentage of area of migration in previously unused culture medium. Test culture media had previously been used for 5 h culture of fragments of jejunal biopsy specimens with and without added alpha-gliadin (0.5 mg/ml). Three coeliac patients on a gluten-free diet are shown as open circles.

accompanied by local delayed hypersensitivity reactions to gluten, (and perhaps to other antigens). Our work on local hypersensitivity in animal models indicates that it is probably the delayed component of the local immune response which causes villous atrophy and crypt hyperplasia in this and other intestinal diseases. However, other immunological and biochemical factors may influence the induction and recall of local CMI reactions, e.g. by enhancing intestinal permeability to food antigens.

ACKNOWLEDGEMENTS

This work has been supported by a grant from the National Fund for Research into Crippling Diseases, and by research facilities supplied by E. Merck Ltd.

References

Asquith, P. (1974). Cell mediated immunity in coeliac disease. In: (W. Th. J. M. Hekkens, and A. S. Pena (eds.) Coeliac Disease, p.242. (Leiden: Stenfert Kroese)

Elves, M. W. and Ferguson, A. (1975). The humoral immune response to allografts of fetal small intestine in mice. Br. J. Exp. Pathol., 56, 454

Ferguson, A. (1973). Implantation of tissue under the kidney capsule. In: Handbook of Experimental Immunology, p.312. (Oxford: Blackwell Scientific Publications)

Ferguson, A. (1974). Lymphocytes in coeliac disease. In: W. Th. J. M. Hekkens, and A. S. Pena (eds.) p.242 Coeliac Disease. (Leiden: Stenfert Kroese)

Ferguson, A. (1976). Coeliac disease and food allergy. In: A. Ferguson and R. N. M. MacSween (eds.) Immunological Aspects of the Liver and the Gastrointestinal Tract. (Lancaster: MTP)

Ferguson, A. and Carswell, F. (1972). Precipitins to dietary proteins in serum and upper intestinal secretions of coeliac children. Br. Med. J., 1, 75

Ferguson, A. and Jarrett, E. E. E. (1975). Hypersensitivity reactions in the small intestine. I Thymus dependence of experimental "partial villous atrophy" Gut, 16, 114

Ferguson, A., MacDonald, T. T., McClure, J. P. and Holden, R. J. (1975). Cell mediated immunity to gliadin within the small intestinal mucosa in coeliac disease. Lancet, i, 895

Ferguson, A. and Murray, D. (1971). Quantitation of intraepithelial lymphocytes in human jejunum. Gut, **14,** 429

Ferguson, A. and Parrott, D. M. V. (1972a). The effects of antigen deprivation on thymus dependent and thymus independent lymphocytes in the small intestine of the mouse. Clin. Exp. Immunol., **12,** 477

Ferguson, A. and Parrott, D. M. V. (1972b). Growth and development of "antigen-free" grafts of foetal mouse intestine. J. Pathol., **106,** 95

Ferguson, A. and Parrott, D. M. V. (1973). Histopathology and time course of rejection of allografts of mouse small intestine. Transplantation, **15,** 546

Guy-Grande, D. Griscelli, C. and Vassalli, P. (1974). The gut associated lymphoid system. Nature and properties of the large dividing cells. Eur. J. Immunol., **4,** 35

Hedberg, C. A., Reiser, S. and Reilly R. W. (1968). Intestinal phase of the runting syndrome in mice. II Observations on nutrient absorption. Transplantation, **12,** 479

Hekkens, W. Th. J. M. and Pena, A. S. (eds.) (1974). Coeliac Disease. (Leiden: Stenfert Kroese)

Holmes, G. K. T., Asquith, P., Stokes, P. L. and Cooke, W. T. (1973). Cellular infiltrate of jejunal biopsies in adult coeliac disease in relation to gluten withdrawal. Gut, **14,** 429

MacDonald, T. T. and Ferguson, A. (1976). Hypersensitivity reactions in the small intestine. II The effects of allograft rejection on mucosal architecture and lymphoid cell infiltrate. Gut, **17,** 81

MacDonald, T. J. and Ferguson, A. (1977). Hypersensitivity reactions in the small intestine. 3. The effects of allograft rejection and of graft-versus-host disease on epithelial cell kinetics. Cell Tiss. Kinet., **10,** 301

Parrot, D. M. V. and Ferguson, A. (1974). Selective migration of lymphocytes within the mouse small intestine. Immunology, **26,** 571

15

Schizophrenia, cereal grains and the gut barrier

Coeliac disease as a model

F. C. DOHAN

INTRODUCTION

The purposes of this paper are: (1) to present a brief summary of the evidence that glutamine, glutamic acid, proline-rich polypeptides from ingested cereal grain glutens play a pathogenic role in the production of schizophrenic symptoms in those hereditarily susceptible to this disorder; (2) to speculate briefly as to the possible role of the gut barrier system in relation to the psychotoxic effects, the hypothesized genetic factors in coeliac disease and schizophrenia, as well as the antigenic nature of the polypeptides. A more comprehensive summary and discussion has been published elsewhere (Dohan, 1978a).

The data have led me to propose the following hypotheses.

HYPOTHESES

I. **Principal hypothesis:** One or more components of cereal grains (and possibly other foods) are the major environmental factor which envokes schizophrenia in those hereditarily susceptible to it.

II. **Subsidiary hypotheses:** (1) one or more of the polypeptides produced by peptic-pancreatic digestion of certain glutamine, proline-rich food proteins (e.g. one or more of those found in glutens of cereal

155

grains) are psychotoxic. (2) They reach the brain of the schizophrenic because the small gut, and possibly other, barrier systems (enzymatic, lysosomal, membranous, immunological, other) suffer defects of an unknown nature. (3) The basic gut barrier defect is due to one or more abnormal genes common to coeliac disease and schizophrenia. (4) The differences in the two diseases are determined largely by the dissimilar components of the genotypes.

SUMMARY OF EVIDENCE

1. Two studies demonstrating highly significant ($p < 0.01$) increases in the rates of improvement in relapsed schizophrenics on a strict cereal grain-free, milk-free diet and the abolition of this effect when wheat gluten was added to the diet without the staff or patients knowing about it (Dohan et al., 1969a, and 1969b; Dohan and Grasberger, 1973).

2. Highly significant worsening of treated schizophrenics ($p < 0.001$) when wheat gluten was added to a cereal grain-free, milk-free diet and their subsequent improvement when administration of gluten was stopped (Singh and Kay, 1976).

3. The production, after a long latent period, of stereotyped and catalepsy-like behaviour in rats by intracerebral injection of glutamine, glutamic acid, proline-rich polypeptides derived from a peptic-pancreatic enzyme digestate of wheat gliadin (Dohan, Levitt, and Kushnir, 1978b).

4. A highly significant positive correlation ($r = 0.96$, $p < 0.01$) between changes in first admissions for schizophrenia and changes in wheat and rye consumption during World War II (Dohan, 1966).

5. Epidemiologic evidence that schizophrenia occurs with apparently lesser frequency (Dohan, 1966), in societies eating mostly or only these cereal grains (e.g. rice, maize, millets, etc.) with lesser content of glutamine and proline than wheat, rye, and barley, the cereal grains usually eliminated in the so called 'gluten-free' diet used in the treatment of coeliac disease.

6. Clinical observations suggesting that schizophrenia and coeliac disease (gluten enteropathy) a familial disorder made symptomatic by ingestion of especially glutamine and proline rich cereal grains, occur in the lifetime of the same individual considerably more frequently than chance expectancy (Graff and Handford, 1961; Dohan, 1970). This suggests the possibility that these two probably polygenic disorders may have one or more, but not all, genes in common.

7. The prominence in adult coeliac patients eating a (gluten-contain-

ing) regular diet of psychiatric symptoms, e.g. apathy, depression, irritability, delusions, paranoid thinking, and psychoses (Paulley, 1959) and, in coeliac children, of stereotyped and schizoid behaviour (Käser, 1961) as well as the rapid improvement in behaviour of coeliacs when started on a 'gluten-free' diet (Townley and Anderson, 1967).

8. The production in many coeliac patients on a 'gluten-free diet' of markedly abnormal, even psychotic behaviour, a few hours after a large oral dose of wheat gluten, or its subfraction, gliadin, or the polypeptides produced by their digestion with pepsin and pancreatic enzymes (Bayless and Cocco, 1969; Rubin et al., 1973; Kowlessar, 1968); as well as evidence 'that glutamine containing peptide is found in the plasma ultrafiltrates of coeliac patients after gliadin ingestion but not in normal subjects' (Kowlessar et al., 1970).

9. The occurrence in schizophrenics during the pre-phenothiazine era, when cereal grain consumption was considerably greater than at present, of metabolic abnormalities and histological changes in the small intestine similar to those now recognized in coeliac patients (references in Dohan and Grasberger, 1973; Dohan, 1976). That similar gut lesions have not been found at autopsy (Dohan, 1969a) or by biopsy (Stevens, et al., 1975; Dean et al., 1975) in present-day schizophrenics suggests that the demonstrated effect of increased cereal grain intake on the production of coeliac gut lesions (Weinstein, 1974) may have played a role (as may have the absence of phenothiazines) in the pathogenesis of the gut changes reported in schizophrenics prior to World War II.

DISCUSSION AND SPECULATIONS

The material presented above provides only circumstantial evidence that glutamine, glutamic acid, proline-rich polypeptides from cereal grain glutens do pass the gut barrier of schizophrenics. However, there is some evidence that, after a large oral dose of gliadin, glutamine containing peptides are found in the blood of coeliacs, but not in that of normal subjects (Kowlessar et al., 1970). This possibility has not been examined in schizophrenics. It needs to be done.

There is little, if any, information concerning the possible mechanisms underlying the apparently psychotoxic effect of cereal grains in schizophrenics. At the present time I feel that the most promising working hypothesis is that some of the polypeptides derived by intra-luminal digestion of cereal grain glutens are psychotoxic and, as a result of genetic factors, pass the gut barrier system in sufficient quantity

157

(compare Hemmings, this volume) to enter the brain and affect its function. (See numbered paragraph 3, above.)

It is not known whether or not the antigenic nature of some gluten polypeptides is a characteristic necessary for the psychotoxic effects in schizophrenics. In coeliac disease, although gluten antigens undoubtedly play a major role in producing the characteristic gut lesions, probably due to genetic factors (see Hekkens and Pena, 1974) there is also no clear evidence that the often marked psychiatric symptoms produced in coeliacs by gluten are due to an immunological reaction.

A comparison of schizophrenia and coeliac disease in regard to hypothesized 'immune response genes' suggests that an abnormal immune response to gluten is **not** necessary for the production of psychiatric symptoms in these diseases. The gene determining HLA-B8 cell surface antigen appears to be closely linked to specific immune response genes determining an 'abnormal' response to certain antigens. The occurrence of the HLA-B8 antigen among schizophrenics is **not** increased (Zmijewski and Dohan, 1976) while it is markedly increased in patients with coeliac disease; yet patients with either disease develop psychiatric symptoms when gluten or its derivatives are given.

However, the genetically determined 'disordered immune response' of coeliacs is probably an important factor determining the intense immune response of their gut mucosa to gluten. On the other hand, schizophrenics, most of whom presumably lack these hypothetical 'immune response genes' may need considerably greater doses of ingested gluten to produce an intense immune response in the gut mucosa. This might account for the coeliac-like changes in the intestines of schizophrenics examined post mortem before World War II when cereal grain consumption was generally much greater than now and the absence of such changes in schizophrenics examined during the past 10 years.

I have hypothesized that one or more genes are common to coeliac disease and schizophrenia and that this gene (or genes) results in a defective gut barrier system for glutamine, glutamic acid, proline-rich peptides. The considerations presented above suggest the product(s) of this common gene (or genes) probably does not determine the enhanced immune response to these peptides. It seems likely that the basic genetic defect in both diseases is at a level (e.g. enzymatic, membranous, lysosomal, other) which permits increased passage of the peptides through the gut barrier and is a necessary precondition for the genetically determined enhanced immune response to these peptides by coeliacs and for the suggestive evidence that on a considerably higher gluten intake schizophrenics may develop coeliac-like gut lesions.

These and other possible mechanisms will deserve consideration if future studies by independent investigators confirm the evidence acquired to date that cereal grains play a pathogenic role in evoking schizophrenic symptoms in those hereditarily susceptible to this disorder.

References

Bayless, T., Cocco, A. Personal communication, 1969

Dean, G., Hanniffy, L., Stevens, F., Temperley, I., O'Broin, J. D. Scott, J., Cahalane, S. F. (1975). Schizophrenia and coeliac disease. J. Irish Med. Assoc., **68**, 545

Dohan, F. C. (1966). Cereals and schizophrenia — data and hypothesis. Acta Psychiat. Scand., **42**, 125

Dohan, F. C. (1969a). Schizophrenia: possible relationship to cereal grains and celiac disease. In: (S. Sankar (ed.) Schizophrenia: Current Concepts and Research. P.539. (Hicksville, N.Y.: P.J.D. Publications Ltd.)

Dohan, F. C., Grasberger, J., Lowell, F., Johnston, Jr., H., Arbegast, A. (1969b). Relapsed schizophrenics: more rapid improvement on a milk and cereal-free diet. Br. J. Psychiat., **115**, 595

Dohan, F. C. (1970). Coeliac disease and schizophrenia (Letter) Lancet, **i**, 897

Dohan, F. C., Grasberger, J. C. (1973). Relapsed schizophrenics: Earlier discharge from the hospital after cereal-free, milk-free diet. Am. J. Psychiat., **130**, 685

Dohan, F. C. (1976a). The possible pathogenic effect of cereal grains in schizophrenia — celiac disease as a model. Acta Neurol. (Napoli), **31**, 195, 1976a.

Dohan, F. C. (1978a). Schizophrenia: are some food-deprived polypeptides pathogenic? In G. P. and W. A. Hemmings (eds.) The Biological Basis of Schizophrenia, Vol. 1 (Lancaster: MTP Press)

Dohan, F. C., Levitt, D., Kushnir, L. (1978b). Abnormal behaviour after intracerebral injection of polypeptides from wheat gliadin. Pavlovian J. Biol. Sci. (in press)

Dohan, F. C., Levitt, D., Kushnir, L. (1976b). Unpublished, 1976b.

Graff, H., Handford, A. (1961). Celiac syndrome in the case history of five schizophrenics. Psychiat. Q., **35**, 306

Hekkens, W. Th. J. M. and Pena, A. S. (eds.) (1974). Coeliac Disease.

Proceedings of the Second International Coeliac Symposium. (Leiden: H. E. Stenfert Kroese.)

Käser, H. (1961). Diagnose und Klinik der Coeliake. Ann. Paediat. (Basel), **197**, 320

Kowlessar, O. D. (1968). Personal communication

Kowlessar, O. D., Warren, R. E., Bronstein, H. D. (1970). Celiac disease: enzyme defect or immune mechanism? In: (G. B. J. Glass (ed.). Progress in Gastroenterology, p.409. (New York: Grune and Stratton)

Paulley, J. W. (1959). Emotion and personality in the etiology of steatorrhea. Am. J. Digest. Dis. **4**, 352

Rubin, C. (1973). Personal communication

Singh, M. M., Kay, S. R. (1976). Wheat gluten as a pathogenic factor in schizophrenia. Science, **191**, 401

Stevens, F. M., Lloyd, R., Geraghty, S., Reynolds, M., Sarsfield, J., Wright, R., McCarthy, C. F. (1975). Proceedings: Schizophrenia and coeliac disease: Is there a positive relationship? Irish J. Med. Sci. **144**, 75

Townley, R. R., Anderson, C. M. (1967). Coeliac disease — a review. Ergebnisse Inn. Med. Kinderheilkunde, **26**, 1

Weinstein, W. M. (1974). Latent celiac sprue. Gastroenterology, **66**, 489

Zmijewski, C., Dohan, F. C. (1976). Unpublished

POSTSCRIPT

Klee and his co-workers have recently reported (Klee, W. A., Zioudrou, C. and Streaty, R. A. (1978) Exorphins-Peptides with opoid activity isolated from wheat gluten and their possible role in the etiology of schizophrenia. In: E. Usdin, (ed.) Endorphins in Mental Health Research. (New York: Macmillan) that a peptide fraction (exorphins), produced by the digestion of wheat gluten (or gliadin) with pepsin alone, has naloxone-reversible endorphin-like activity in their **in vitro** test systems, while another fraction antagonizes these effects. The peptides in both fractions deserve careful study because of the well known behavioural effects of endorphins and other brain peptides. The authors point out that the peptides in both fractions are very hydrophobic, and show a pre-dominance of leucine and isoleucine and contain phenylalanine and tyrosine but almost no charged amino acids. They suggest that such peptides 'might be expected to traverse biological membranes, including the blood brain barrier with relative ease'. Thus, investigators of the psychotoxic effects of gluten and gliadin peptides and their passage across the gut barrier should direct this attention not only to the most common (Glutamine-glutamic acid-proline rich) peptides produced during digestion but also to unusual peptides such as those described by Klee and his associates.

16

The chemistry of gliadin

A. L. PATEY

INTRODUCTION

Becarri, in 1745, and Einhof, in 1805, were the first to study the proteins present in wheat flour, but the name 'gliadin' was not known until 1820 when Taddei used this name to describe the alcohol-soluble protein components of flour. Since then, an ever-increasing amount of literature has appeared on gliadin. Up to 1970, Chemical Abstracts quotes 536 references on the subject, however, in the last 8 years, over 180 more articles have appeared.

But why have the gliadins been the subject of so much research? The answer to this question is that a knowledge of the properties of the gliadins is required by workers in many unrelated medical and scientific disciplines. Thus, gliadin proteins are investigated by the baking technologist for it is the quality and quantity of protein that helps to give wheat flour its characteristic baking properties (Pomeranz, 1968). Gliadins interest the gastroenterologist for wheat protein contains the toxic factor associated with coelic disease (Evans and Patey, 1974), this being discovered by Dicke only in 1950. The psychiatrist is fascinated by the thought that wheat proteins may act as pathogenic factors in schizophrenia (Singh and Kay, 1976), while the biochemist displays his interest with, for example, gliadin absorption into mammalian tissues (C. Hemmings et al., 1976a, b). To the chemist, the attractions of the gliadins are their unusual structural properties and this is the subject of this paper.

FLOUR PROTEIN

Classification of protein

The major constituents of wheat flour, which is the milled endosperm of the grain, are starch (about 70-75%), moisture (about 10-15%), protein (about 8-6%) together with lipids (about 1-2%). There are also trace amounts of other materials such as nucleic acids.

Flour protein consists of four heterogeneous groups, as classified by Osborne in 1907. Flour albumins are soluble in water, globulins in dilute salt solutions, glutenins in dilute alkali and gliadins in aqueous alcohol. The first two groups are present in only small amounts with respect to total flour protein, while the glutenins (of high molecular weight and very heterogeneous) have poor solubility characteristics and, thus, have not been extensively studied.

By far the most important grouping of flour proteins are the gliadins which make up about 40-45% of total flour protein. The gliadins have been investigated in detail for about 70 years and published reports have been reviewed extensively (Osborne, 1907; Blish, 1945; Kasarda et al., 1971; Patey, 1972; Patey, 1974).

Chemistry of gliadin

The gliadins fall into four groups (α, β, γ and ω) with respect to mobility upon starch-gel electrophoresis at pH 3.2, with the α-gliadins having the fastest mobility and the ω-gliadins the slowest (Kasarda et al., 1971). By combinations of ion-exchange chromatography and electrophoresis, as many as three α, four β, three γ and six to eight ω-components have been identified in individual flours, but each variety of flour has a different set of individual proteins. For example, one of the four β-gliadins occurring in a certain flour could be unique to the wheat from which it was made.

The standard method of isolation of the gliadins from flour is by dilute acetic acid or 70% ethanol extraction of butanol-defatted flour, followed by carboxymethyl — (Patey and Evans, 1973) or sulphoethyl-cellulose (Platt and Kasarda, 1971) chromatography. Since the gliadins are very resistant to denaturation (Shearer et al., 1975), these operations can be carried out at room temperature. Gel filtration is used to rid the gliadins (especially α-gliadins) of high molecular weight contaminants. The amount of carbohydrate associated with the gliadins, so prepared, has been estimated as being equivalent to one molecule of monosaccharide for every ten of protein (Bernardin et al., 1976). In other words, gliadins are not true glycoproteins and any sugar which may be present in a preparation is probably due to contamination from, for example, dextran gels. It is most essential to start with a pure flour milled from a single wheat variety if individual proteins are to be isolated easily. Much biochemical/medical research is made more difficult than it should be, if the gliadin used is prepared from commercially-obtained blends of flours which contain countless different proteins (Patey, 1973).

The molecular weights of α, β and γ-gliadins are consistently between 32 000 and 44 000 by sodium dodecyl sulphate polyacrylamide gel electrophoresis (Bietz and Wall, 1972; Hamauzu et al., 1972; Ewart, 1973) but reported molecular weights vary considerably and are generally much higher when older techniques are used. ω-Gliadins have molecular weights roughly double (around 70 000) those of other gliadins and are the minor component (about 10%) of the gliadin mixture. The ω-gliadins have also been named athins (Booth and Ewart, 1969), as they contain no sulphur amino-acids, although this name is not in general usage.

The α, β and γ-gliadins (each about 30% of the gliadin mixture) have been shown usually to have single polypeptide chains and display intramolecular disulphide bonding (Stevens, 1973), although there is some evidence (Patey and Waldron, 1976) of possibly more than one chain being present in certain gliadins. The amino-acid composition of a typical gliadin (Maris Widgeon wheat α_2-gliadin) is displayed in Table 1 (Patey and Waldron, 1976). As can be seen there is about 40% of glutamic acid (mostly as glutamine) and about 15% proline: gliadins are the only proteins that contain a high proportion of glutamine and proline. In nutritional terms, there is a deficiency in lysine, arginine and histidine. Proteins from different varieties of wheat afford similar analyses to Maris Widgeon α_2-gliadin but with small distinct differences. As an example, Gold Seal wheat α_{1B}-gliadin differs from α_{1C}-by 7 residues and from α_2-by 9 residues in a total of 265 (Kasarda et al., 1971). The high content of proline in the gliadins is a contributing factor towards the average α-helix content being 38% as shown by circular dichroism and optical rotatory dispersion experiments (Cluskey and Wu, 1971).

Only in the last four years have sequence studies been performed on gliadin proteins. Many hundreds of complete protein sequences are now known as are many thousands of partial sequences, but the reason that

Table 1 Nearest integer residues per minimal molecular weight (assuming lys is unity); Maris Widgeon α_2-gliadin

Asp	4	Met	2
Thr	7	Ile	4
Ser	18	Leu	11
Glu	73	Tyr	4
Pro	38	Phe	9
Gly	5	Lys	1
Ala	5	His	2
½ Cys	6	Arg	3
Val	5	Trp	1

wheat proteins have lagged behind in being sequenced is that the complex nature of the gliadin mixture has, until recently, made it very difficult to isolate even milligramme quantities of pure proteins. However, several pure α- and γ-gliadins have now been isolated. Table 2 shows the first twelve amino-acid residues of an α-gliadin of Gold Seal wheat (Kasarda et al., 1974) and a γ-gliadin of Kolibri wheat (Patey et al., 1975). Seven of the first twelve residues are identical. In a further study (Bietz et al., 1977), two Ponca wheat γ-gliadins have been partially sequenced. One was identical in N-terminal sequence to Gold Seal α-gliadin, the other completely different. When one considers the similarities in amino-acid analyses and N-terminal sequences between the α- and γ-gliadins and also the closeness of many patterns in peptide-mapping studies (Kasarda et al., 1971) of pepsin/trypsin hydrolysed gliadins, there is considerable evidence for there being large regions of polypeptide chain identical in the different proteins. Again, this is evidence that gliadin proteins have evolved from a common precursor protein. Also, it is apparent that the present nomenclature system for gliadins is in need of revision.

Table 2 N-terminal sequences of gliadin proteins

Kolibri γ	$_2$HN-VAL- ILE-VAL-GLN-VAL-ARG-GLN-LEU-GLN-VAL GLN-GLN-
Gold Seal α	$_2$HN-VAL-ARG-VAL-PRO-VAL-PRO-GLN-LEU-GLN-PRO-GLN-ASN-
	1 2 3 4 5 6 7 8 9 10 11 12

CONCLUSION

Research on the chemistry of gliadin seems centred at present on evolving better ways of preparing large amounts of pure proteins with the object of submitting these to N-terminal sequencing and other characterisation studies. No β- or ω-gliadin has been studied in this way. Until further sequencing is performed we can only speculate as to what sort of relationship exists among gliadin components. When we have this information, a better system of nomenclature will most probably be devised (possibly on a molecular weight basis): the present system based on electrophoretic mobility alone is clearly inadequate.

References

Becarri, (1745). De Bononiensi Scientiarium et Artium Instituto atque Academia. Commentarii, **2**, 122

Bernardin, J. E., Saunders, R. M. and Kasarda, D. D. (1976). Absence of carbohydrate in celiac-toxic A-gliadin. Cereal Chem., **53**, 612

Bietz, J. A. and Wall, J. S. (1972). Wheat gluten subunits. Molecular weight determination by SDS polyacrylamide gel electrophoresis. Cereal Chem., **49**, 416

Bietz, J. A., Huebner, F. R., Sanderson, J. E. and Wall, J. S. (1977). Wheat gliadin homology revealed through N-terminal amino acid sequence analysis. Cereal Chem., **54**, 1070

Blish, M. J. (1945). Wheat gluten. Adv. Protein Chem., **2**, 337

Booth, M. R. and Ewart, J. A. D. (1969). Studies on four components of wheat gliadins. Biochem. Biophys. Acta, **181**, 226

Cluskey, J. E. and Wu, Y. V. (1971). Optical rotatory dispersion, circular dichroism, and infra red studies of wheat gluten proteins in various solvents. Cereal Chem., **48**, 203

Dicke, W. K. (1950). Coeliakie. Een ouderzoek naar de nadelige invloed van sommige graansoorten op de lijder aan coeliakie. MD Thesis, Utrecht

Einhof, H. (1805). J.Der Chemie, **5**, 131

Evans, D. J. and Patey, A. L. (1974). Chemistry of wheat proteins and the nature of the damaging substances. Clin. Gastroenterol., **3**(I), 199

Ewart, J. A. D. (1973). SDS-electrophoresis of wheat gliadins. J. Sci. Food Agric., **24**, 685

Hamauzu, Z., Arakawa, T. and Yonezawa, D. (1972). Molecular

weights of glutenin and gliadin polypeptides estimated by SDS gel electrophoresis. Agric. Biol. Chem., **36**, 1829

Hemmings, C., Hemmings, W. A. and Patey, A. L. (1976a). The fate of oral doses of α-gliadin in suckling and adult rats. IRCS Med. Sci., **4**, 38

Hemmings, C., Hemmings, W. A. and Patey, A. L. (1976b). The fate of oral doses of β-and γ-gliadin in adult rats. IRCS Med. Sci., **4**, 152

Kasarda, D. D., Nimmo, C. C. and Kohler, G. O. (1971). Proteins and the amino-acid composition of wheat fractions. Wheat Chemistry and Technology, A.A.C.A., 227

Kasarda, D. D., DaRoza, D. A. and Ohms, J. I. (1974). N-terminal sequence of α_2-gliadin. Biochim. Biophys. Acta, **351**, 290

Osborne, T. B. (1907). The proteins of wheat kernel

Patey, A. L. (1972). Some basic isothiocyanates and investigation on gliadin. Ph.D. Thesis, London

Patey, A. L. and Evans, D. J. (1973). Large-scale preparation of gliadin proteins. J. Sci. Food Agric., **24**, 1229

Patey, A. L. (1973). Toxic component of wheat gluten. Lancet, ii, 1096

Patey, A. L. (1974). Gliadin: the protein mixture toxic to coeliac patients. Lancet, i, 722

Patey, A. L., Evans, D. J., Tiplady, R., Byfield, P.G.H. and Matthews, E.W. (1975). Sequence comparison of γ-gliadin and coeliac-toxic α-gliadin. Lancet, ii, 718

Patey, A. L. and Waldron, N. M. (1976). Gliadin proteins from Maris Widgeon wheat. J. Sci. Food Agric., **27**, 838

Platt, S. G. and Kasarda, D. D. (1971). Separation and characterization of α-gliadin fractions. Biochim. Biophys. Acta, **243**, 407

Pomeranz, Y. (1968). Relation between chemical composition and bread-making potentialities of wheat flour. Adv. Food Res., **16**, 335

Shearer, G., Patey, A. L. and McWeeny, D. J. (1975). Wheat flour proteins: the selectivity of solvents and the stability of the gliadin and glutenin fractions of stored flours. J. Sci. Food Agric., **26**, 337

Singh, M. M. and Kay, S. R. (1976). Wheat gluten as a pathogenic factor in schizophrenia. Science, **191**, 401

Stevens, D. J. (1973). Reaction of wheat protein with sulphite.III. Measurement of labile and reactive bonds in gliadin and in the protein aleurone cells. J. Sci. Food Agric., **24**, 279

Taddei, G. (1820). Annals of Philosophy, **15**, 390

17

Urticaria and dietary hypersensitivity

A. M. DENMAN, T. PLATTS-MILLS, P. J. BRERETON, L. DODDYMEAD, R. SOAN, B. K. PELTON, G. LOEWI, M. SHINER and D. K. PETERS

INTRODUCTION

The concept of dietary hypersensitivity once highly fashionable in medical circles, spas and watering places was soon derided when the era of scientific investigation in medicine opened. Nevertheless such theories have gained fresh respectability with the introduction of precise techniques for measuring antibodies to immunogenic constituents of the diet. The unequivocal demonstration of gluten hypersensitivity in coeliac disease has aroused suspicions that other antigens may induce similar disorders albeit less florid in their mode of presentation. Moreover dietary hypersensitivity has been incriminated in a wide range of chronic gastrointestinal diseases appearing for the first time in societies which are in the process of adopting a highly sophisticated standard of living, including a change in dietary habits. Indeed other diseases now endemic in developed countries such as myocardial infarction have been attributed to dietary antigens (Davies et al., 1974). Whilst such claims may often have been exaggerated, the striking discrepancy between the incidence of certain diseases in relatively primitive communities and in advanced, urban societies draws attention to the possible importance of environmental factors including dietary ones. A noteworthy example is the paucity of inflammatory arthritis, and in particular rheumatoid arthritis, in rural populations of Bantu Africans (Beighton et al., 1975).

167

The explosive onset of disseminated lupus erythematosus in Jamaican negroes and in the coloured population of the United States emphasizes the vulnerability of people from diverse races to new diseases when their social conditions are drastically distorted.

Chronic urticaria is a common disease of the skin consisting of ephemeral lesions of variable size which have the characteristics of an acute hypersensitivity reaction mediated by histamine release. The onset is often sudden and the disease follows a variable course commonly persisting for several years. The tongue, glottis and peri-orbital tissues are commonly involved and there is no evidence that such features indicate a different pathogenesis. We have been impressed by the number of Ugandan immigrants referred to this Centre who have acquired the disease soon after their arrival from East Africa although no formal analysis of its incidence has yet been completed. A range of possibilities must be considered. Thus, skin reactions are provoked by hypersensitivity to black flies or their products in immigrant populations when first resident in the Altamira region of Brazil (Pinheiro et al., 1974) emphasizing the wide range of possible factors which must be taken into consideration. We have analysed the association between chronic urticaria and dietary hypersensitivity for the following reasons. Firstly a dietary aetiology has long been recognized in a proportion of such patients. Secondly the transient nature of the lesions makes clinical assessment of the disease course very simple and attempts to alter this by dietary exclusion or other therapeutic manoeuvres can readily be monitored. Finally, biopsies are obtainable without difficulty for histological or immunochemical analysis. Thus chronic urticaria is a good working model for examining the immuno-pathological consequences of common environmental antigens.

MATERIALS AND METHODS

Patients

Fifty four patients with chronic urticaria were investigated who fulfilled the following criteria.

(1) Characteristic skin lesions had appeared over a period of at least 3 months.

(2) The lesions were promptly suppressed by anti-histamine drugs.

(3) No evidence of systemic disease was present to which the urticaria may have been secondary. β-1-C esterase inhibitor deficiency was as far as routinely possible excluded by detecting this protein immuno-

phoretically in patients' serum although functional tests of its activity were not conducted.

Laboratory investigations

These were performed in all or a high proportion of the patients.

Immunoglobulins

IgG, IgA and IgM levels were determined by immunodiffusion and total and specific IgE values by radioallergosorbant tests.

Complement

Total haemolytic activity (CH50) was measured using sheep erythrocytes as indicator cells. C3 conversion products were sought by two-dimensional immunoelectrophoresis.

Immune complexes

Sera were screened for immune complexes firstly by exposure to fresh granulocytes which were thereafter stained with fluorescein-labelled anti-human Ig antisera for phagocytosed Ig and secondly for evidence of anti-complementary activity.

Standard techniques were used for these measurements.

Lymphocyte function in vitro

Lymphocyte transformation by phytohaemagglutinin (PHA), Concanavalin A (Con A) and pokeweed mitogen (PWM) were measured by carbon-14 thymidine incorporation using cultures of 0.2×10^6 cells in microtitre plates.

Lymphocytes with receptors for sheep red cells and with surface Ig detectable by immunofluorescence were also enumerated.

The techniques were those routinely adopted in clinical immunology laboratories.

Skin biopsies

These were examined by light microscopy using appropriate stains for the

Table 1 Elimination diet

Diet	I	II	III	IV
Cereals	rice	Ryvita	potatoes	—
Meat	lamb	chicken	beef	—
Vegetables	lettuce	cabbage	tomato	carrots
Fruit	oranges	apricots	grapefruit	—
Fats	olive oil	margarine	margarine	—
Dairy products	—	—	milk	cheese milk
Misc.	salt	syrup	jam	sugar

Notes. 1. This is not the full list, but is abbreviated to illustrate the kind of rotation which is used.
2. Tinned and preserved foods should be withheld initially.
3. Each diet is adopted for one to four weeks, depending on the clinical response, the order of rotation being determined by the initial history.

detection of mast cells and basophils and by indirect immunofluorescence for Ig and complement deposits.

Other tests were performed on selected patients as will be indicated in the text.

Exclusion diets

Initially a series of sequential diets was adopted by which each major group of potentially sensitizing foods was excluded in turn (Table 1). This was better tolerated by patients than more stringent diets but often gave equivocal results.

For the major part of this study, therefore, one of two policies was adopted. When symptoms were sufficiently severe and this arrangement was socially practicable, patients were admitted to hospital and maintained on fluids alone reinforced with vitamins and glucose for up to one week. At this stage they were placed on a less restricted diet (Table 2) which nevertheless excluded most potential allergens. Patients who had not first been admitted for a period of complete dietary deprivation embarked on this basic diet from the outset. The patients were provided

Table 2 Basic exclusion diet: principal features

Permitted	Major exclusions
Fresh fruit and vegetables	Meat and poultry
Fresh fruit juice	Eggs
Tea, coffee, sugar	Milk and dairy products
Rice	Tinned, frozen and preserved food
Gluten free bread	Bread, biscuits, cake, flour
Olive oil	
Barley sugar	
Tomor margarine	

with standard diary sheets to record the frequency and severity of urticarial attacks.

Once a remission had been induced, excluded items were restored sequentially to the diet. Frequent visits to the Clinic and Dietetics Department enabled patients' progress to be followed and the diet to be adjusted accordingly. Three months was regarded as the shortest period necessary before abandoning treatment in patients who failed to respond.

Table 3 urticaria — principal causes

1) **Drugs** — penicillin; salicylates
2) **Therapeutic agents** — hormones
3) **Infections** — viruses
4) **Systemic disease** — thyroid disease
5) **Pollens**
6) **Dietary** — (a) **Natural** — milk, cheese
   eggs
   nuts
   chocolate
   cereals
   fruits
   (b) **Additives** – penicillin
   yeast
   aliphatic aldehydes
   azo-dyes
   benzoic acids

171

Table 4 Analysis of patients with chronic urticaria

Preceding infection	13
Exclusion diet attempted	27
other	14
Total	**54**

RESULTS

Incidence of dietary hypersensitivity

The aetiology of chronic urticaria has been admirably reviewed (Warin and Champion, 1974) and the principal causes are summarized in Table 3 which emphasizes the most important dietary causes of this disorder.

We have studied 54 patients of whom 32 were female and 22 male and whose age ranged from 3 to 60 years. In six of these patients joint symptoms characteristic of serum sickness arthritis were a prominent clinical feature but these did not fulfil the accepted criteria of 'definite' or 'classical' rheumatoid arthritis (Table 4).

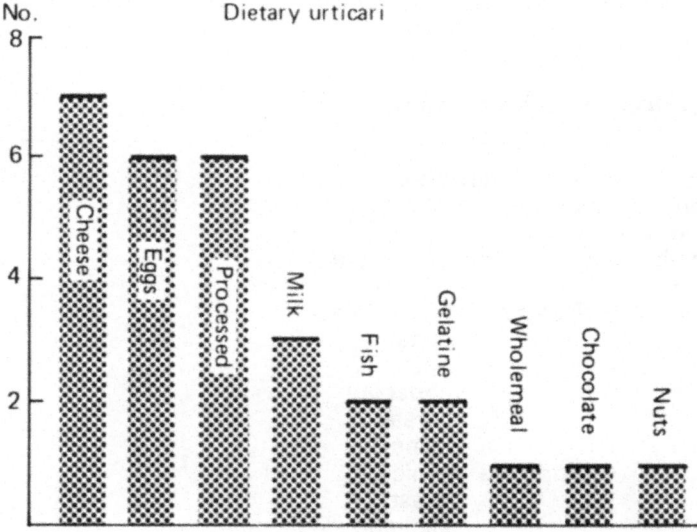

Figure 1 Dietary urticaria. Items responsible for chronic urticaria in 20 patients responding to an exclusion diet

172

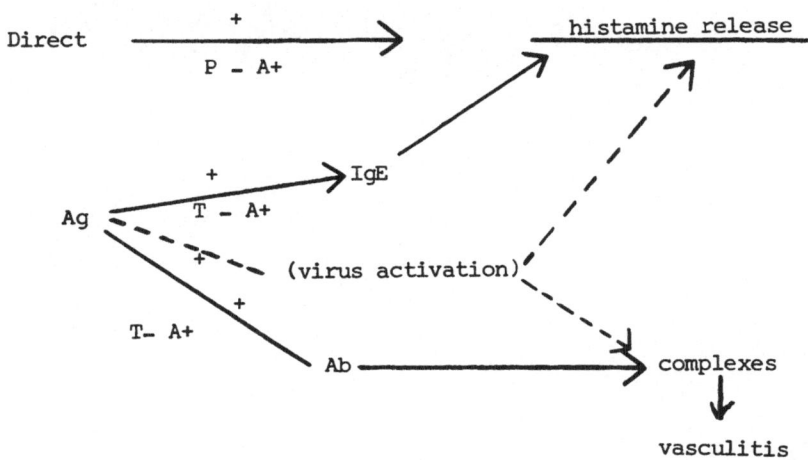

Figure 2 Urticaria: possible mechanism. + = facilitatory factors; — = inhibitory factors; A = gastrointestinal absorption; P = Pharmacological factors; T = T-lymphocyte suppressor populations; Ag = antigen; Ab = antibody

In 13 patients the onset of urticaria was preceded by a clear history of a severe infectious episode mostly characteristic of a virus infection of the respiratory tract. An exclusion diet was instituted in 27 patients and of these 20 responded, mostly within the first 3 weeks of treatment. The dietary items which were responsible are indicated in Figure 1. Since 29 items are recorded, it is apparent that patients were commonly sensitive to more than one dietary constituent. The preponderance of cheese and eggs is also evident.

Analysis of pathogenesis

The possible mechanisms by which dietary agents may induce urticaria are outlined in Figure 2 which forms the basis for analysing the results of tests performed in our own laboratory and by other groups.

Direct mechanisms

Although histamine release explains both the clinical and histological features of chronic urticaria, it is not certain that immunological

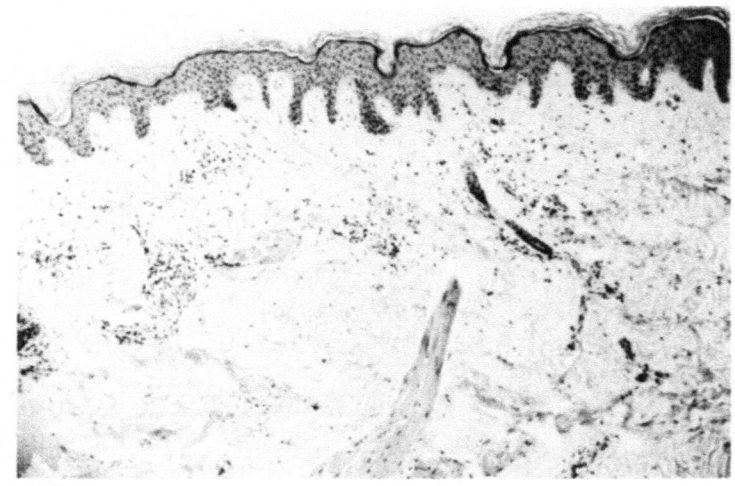

Figure 3A

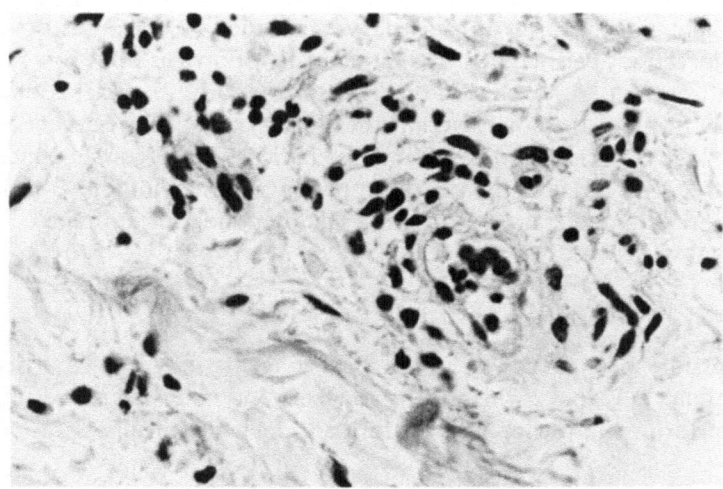

Figure 3 Urticaria: skin biopsy. Toluidine Blue stain; (A) × 150; (B) × 1200. The biopsy was taken from an active lesion but clinically normal skin showed essentially the same changes.

mechanisms are responsible. Indeed IgE coated basophils from such patients appear to release less histamine than those from normal subjects after challenge with antigen, in this instance anti-IgE antiserum (Greaves et al., 1974) suggesting that the abnormality may be primarily pharmacological. Nor has the possibility been investigated that the responsible items are absorbed in excessive amounts.

Immunological mechanisms

Acute hypersensitivity

The similarities between atopic disorders such as allergic rhinitis and chronic urticaria immediately suggests that the latter also is mediated by reaginic IgE antibody (Figure 3). Specific IgE antibodies to food antigens have been reportedly detected by radioimmunoassay (Hoffman and Haddad, 1974). In our series levels of total IgE antibody were slightly elevated in two patients but otherwise normal whilst the presence of specific IgE antibody to the responsible antigens has not yet been confirmed. Similarly skin tests for both immediate and delayed hypersensitivity have given inconclusive results.

Response to disodium cromoglycate

Disodium cromoglycate effectively blocks many forms of acute hypersensitivity by interfering with histamine release from basophils sensitized with IgE. The symptoms of milk protein intolerance in infants have been prevented by this drug (Freiser and Berger, 1973). In our experience, disodium cromoglycate suppresses the skin reactions of some forms of food allergy including those in which these are exacerbated by physical factors such as pressure, sunlight, short periods of exposure to ultra-violet irradiation or cold.

An example of this blockade is summarized in Figure 4 which portrays the findings in a patient with gastrointestinal allergy. This 53-year-old lady gave a history of severe urticaria and anaphylactic symptoms whenever she ate fish or gelatine-containing food. She was also sensitive to penicillin. Numerous skin tests were positive and that to house-dust was particularly strong. The jejunal biopsy before treatment was normal. Instillation of gelatine into the jejunum induced a severe clinical reaction and epithelial changes by both light and immunofluorescence microscopy. She received disodium cromoglycate by mouth both before and during a second challenge with gelatine and on this occasion the clinical symptoms were suppressed whilst the changes in the jejunum were not exacerbated. There were no disturbances of serum Ig levels nor any abnormality in the distribution of Ig staining cells in the jejunum by immunofluorescence.

The efficacy of disodium cromoglycate in chronic urticaria is currently the subject of a double-blind controlled trial at this centre.

Impaired control mechanisms

Exaggerated responses to dietary and other allergens have been attributed to impaired control mechanisms and, in particular, to defects in suppressor populations of T lymphocytes. Assays for this function

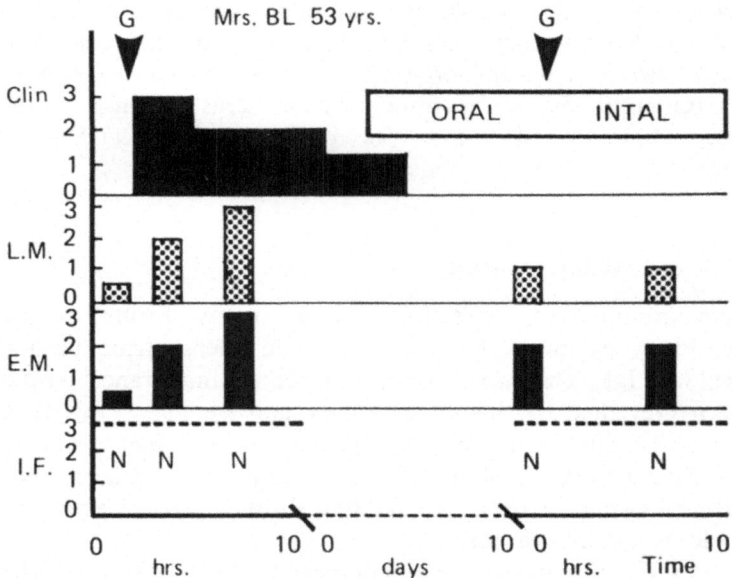

Figure 4 Gastrointestinal allergy blocked by disodium chromoglycate. Clin = clinical symptoms of urticaria and anaphylaxis graded 1 to 3. L.M. = light microscopic findings, i.e. oedema, inflammatory changes and distortion of villi graded 1 to 3. E.M. = electron microscopic findings, i.e. mast cell infiltration and degranulation graded 1 to 3. IF = immunofluorescent changes graded 1 to 3. Interrupted line indicates upper limit of normality. N = normal finding for all classes of Ig staining cells. ▼ = instillation of gelatine. Oral intal = 300 mg disodium cromoglycate three times daily.

with human blood lymphocytes are clearly imperfect; with this reservation lymphocyte function judged by response to standard mitogens and by tests for recognized sub-populations was entirely normal.

IgA deficiency has also been incriminated in the pathogenesis of dietary hypersensitivity but this was not evident in our patients either from serum analysis or immunofluorescence staining of jejunal biopsies.

Immune complex formation

With one exception Ig or complement was not detected in skin biopsies of lesions or uninvolved skin by immunofluorescence. There has been no obvious abnormality in the numbers of Ig staining cells in the jejunum and complement has not been found in this site by immunofluorescence. Furthermore, circulating immune complexes have not been found in the sera of the majority of patients; however the limitations of current techniques for revealing all categories of soluble complex are well recognized. Similarly complement abnormalities have generally been lacking.

Nevertheless evidence of complement activation and soluble complexes in the serum has appeared in two patients with dietary hypersensitivity. Furthermore C3 breakdown products were also detected. The findings in one such patient are outlined in Table 5 and the findings in two

Table 5

Mrs. H. S. aged 55 years
aged 49   rheumatoid arthritis
aged 53   chronic urticaria

exclusion diet: sensitive to cheese and preserved or processed foods
other sensitivities: African violet, thiazide diuretics

Investigations:
initially: no abnormality
aged 55:   developed immune complex glomerulonephritis and complement activation

Clq, C2, C4, C3 — **reduced**
C3 catabolism — **increased**
split C3 products — **present**
properdin factor B; inhibitors — **normal**

Figure 5 Urticaria: split complement products. Two dimensional immunoelectrophoresis on (a) normal serum (b) patient's serum. The arrow denotes the split product.

dimensional immunoelectrophoresis of her serum are illustrated in Figure 5.

The possibility should be considered that immune complex vasculitis makes a major contribution to tissue damage in dietary urticaria, but that the available techniques are too insensitive to detect this process in the majority of patients. Immunopathological studies of patients lacking overt renal disease have not been reported and would be ethically unjustified. The association between urticaria and hypocomplementaemia is now well recognized (Sissons et al., 1974) and should lead to closer scrutiny of such patients for abnormalities of this nature which are not clinically obvious.

Virus activation

Urticaria is commonly associated with acute virus infections. Furthermore such infections may induce hypersensitivity to specific drugs (Green, 1974). The most pertinent example of this interaction is the temporary hypersensitivity to ampicillin seen in patients with infectious mononucleosis who inappropriately receive this antibiotic. The mechanism is unknown but suggests the possibility that persistent infection could account for the sudden onset of dietary hypersensitivity in previously normal people. Such a hypothesis is hard to prove and direct evidence in man is still lacking.

DISCUSSION

A dietary cause has been firmly established in a large proportion of patients with chronic urticaria. At first sight it seems unreasonable to incriminate a single allergen in any one patient (Speer, 1975). However, multiple sensitivity may be too readily accepted as the most common finding since a persistent urticarial reaction to one dietary antigen may well predispose the patient to exacerbations produced by other agents including physical insults. Moreover urticaria for which no obvious cause is found by a relatively short trial of exclusion diets may well need a much longer trial as has been demonstrated in dermatitis herpetiformis provoked by hypersensitivity to gluten (Fry et al., 1973).

The precise mechanism by which dietary hypersensitivity induces chronic urticaria has not been defined and will be hard to analysed until the responsible allergens are available in highly purified form; this requirement has been amply borne out in studies of allergic rhinitis caused by ragweed hypersensitivity. Simple items common to dairy products, beef and eggs are antibiotics which might potentiate hypersensitivity initiated by their therapeutic administration but this possibility has not yet been substantiated in our series.

It is unclear whether dietary antigens which induce chronic urticaria invariably provoke a hypersensitivity reaction in the gastrointestinal tract as well as in the skin and mucous membranes. Undoubtedly, abdominal symptoms and eosinophilic infiltration of the gastric mucous membrane are on occasion the sole manifestations of dietary hypersensitivity (Klein et al., 1970). In addition, hypersensitivity to milk proteins has been responsible for a syndrome of protein losing gastroenteropathy with eosinophilia and retardation of growth (Waldmann et al., 1967). We have recently seen a 9-year-old boy with anaemia, hypoalbuminaemia, a blood eosinophil count of $2200/\mu l$ and a high turnover rate of albumin and transferrin due to protein losing enteropathy. Skin testing to egg was strongly positive and a test meal of eggs induced vomiting, abdominal pain and urticaria. However, such findings are not characteristic of most patients with gastrointestinal allergy and chronic urticaria. There are three major possibilities which would explain the relation of the gut to dietary urticaria.

(1) Qualitative or quantitative differences in the absorption of potential allergens determine the onset of hypersensitivity reactions. That the amount absorbed needs to be considered is illustrated by the widespread liability to lactose intolerance if sufficient milk is consumed

(Bayless et al., 1975). There is insufficient evidence available to evaluate this possibility.

(2) Potential allergens are regularly absorbed and hypersensitivity is genetically determined in a manner analogous with allergens absorbed through the respiratory tract or which induce contact sensitivity. The pattern of immunopathological events, namely immediate hypersensitivity, strongly suggests this but there are hints that other mechanisms account for the disease features, at least in a proportion of patients.

(3) Hypersensitivity involves primarily the gut and lesions at other sites are entirely secondary, for example through the generation of soluble complexes (Doe et al., 1973). At present this suggestion seems true of only a small minority of patients with chronic urticaria but it clearly needs further assessment.

ACKNOWLEDGEMENTS

We are most grateful to Dr. Harold Wilson for his generous help in referring patients for study and to Dr. A. S. Tavill for permission to refer to his unpublished data in his patient with protein losing enteropathy.

References

Bayless, T. M., Rothfeld, B., Massa, C., Wise, L., Paige D. and Bedine, M. S. (1975). Lactose and milk intolerance: clinical implications. N. Engl. J. Med., **292**, 1156

Beighton, P., Solomon, L. and Valkenburg, H. A. (1975). Rheumatoid arthritis in a rural South African Negro population. Ann. Rheum. Dis. **34**, 136

Davies, D. F., Johnson, A. P., Rees, B. W. G., Elwood, P. C. and Abernethy, M. (1974). Food antibodies and myocardial infarction. Lancet, **i**, 1012

Doe, W. F., Booth, C. C. and Brown, D. L. (1973). Evidence for complement-binding immune complexes in adult coeliac disease, Crohn's disease and ulcerative colitis. Lancet, **i**, 402

Freier, S. and Berger, H. (1973). Disodium cromoglycate in gastrointestinal protein intolerance. Lancet, **i**, 913

Fry, L., Seah, P. P., Riches, D. J. and Hoffbrand, A. V (1973). Clearance of skin lesions in dermatitis herpetiformis after glutin withdrawal. Lancet, **i**, 288

Greaves, M. W., Plummer, V. M., McLaughlan, P. and Stanworth,

D. R. (1974). Serum and cell bound IgE in chronic urticaria. Clin. Allergy, **4**, 265

Green, R. H. (1974). The association of viral activation with penicillin toxicity in guinea pigs and hamsters. Yale J. Biol. Med., **3**, 166

Hoffman, D. R. and Haddad, Z. H. (1974). Diagnosis of IgE-mediated reactions to food antigens by radioimmunoassay. J. Allergy Clin. Immunol., **54**, 165

Klein, N. C., Hargrove, R. L., Sleisenger, M. H. and Jeffries, G. H. (1970). Eosinophilic gastroenteritis. Medicine, **49**, 299

Pinheiro, F. P., Bensabath, G., Costa, D., Maroja, O. M., Lins, Z. S. and Andrade, A. H. P. (1974). Haemorrhagic syndrome of Altamira. Lancet, **i**, 639

Sissons, J. G. P., Williams, D. G., Peters, D. K., Boulton-Jones, J. M. and Goldsmith, H. J. (1974). Skin lesions, angio-oedema and hypocomplementaemia. Lancet, **ii**, 1350

Speer, F. (1975). Multiple food allergy. Ann. Allergy, **34**, 71

Waldmann, T. A., Wochner, R. D., Laster, L. and Gordon, R. S. (1967). Allergic gastroenteropathy: a cause of excessive gastro-enteropathy: a cause of excessive gastrointestinal protein loss. N. Engl. J. Med., **276**, 761

Warin, R. and Champion, R. (1974). Major Problems in Dermatology. Vol. I. Urticaria, pp.33-73. (London: W. B. Saunders)

POSTSCRIPT

A double-bind controlled trial of oral disodium cromoglycate (Intal) has now been completed in conjunction with Drs. P. Kingsley and A. M. Edwards. 27 patients with chronic, idiopathic urticaria received 300 mg t.d.s. of the drug or placebo each for a period of 1 month. Each period was followed by a further control period of 1 month during which the patients received neither disodium cromoglycate or placebo. The patients kept a daily record of the frequency and severity of their symptoms and clinical and laboratory examinations were carried out at monthly intervals. No significant differences between the effects of disodium cromoglycate or placebo were observed in terms of the clinical course or laboratory findings in chronic urticaria.

18

A review of endotoxin and its absorption from the gut

E. N. WARDLE

My role today will be to review the clinical significance of endotoxin absorption from the gut and to expose the problem, to which we do not yet know the answer . . . how is endotoxin able to cross the gut mucosa?

The endotoxins of Gram negative bacteria all have a similar structure. At one end of the tripartite molecule is an O-specific polysaccharide which is made up of repeating oligosaccharide units, in the middle is the common core polysaccharide and the really toxic end of the molecule is known as lipid A. This lipid A includes the fatty acids, lauric, myristic and palmitic acids attached to hydroxyl and amino groups on glucosamine. The lipid A is the part which attaches the molecule to the phospholipid of cell membranes. The overall action of endotoxin can be one of total destruction and in this respect the analogy of structure to a nuclear warhead is quite appropriate. The molecular weight is one million but it can be broken into units of 400 000 daltons size which still show biological activity.

The molecule can enter the circulation directly from foci of Gram negative sepsis but we are now also aware that it can enter the portal circulation from the bowel in states of shock, as a result of other types of bowel ischaemia and in certain types of liver disease. One therefore has to consider carefully what factors increase the permeability of the gut mucosa, of the colon in particular, and what mechanisms obviate the normal protective effect of the reticuloendothelial system? The protective cells include the von Kupffer cells of the liver and the phagocytic cells of the spleen. However it should be realized that initial contact with endotoxin tends to inhibit these cells: it is only in animals with endotoxin tolerance that the RES cells are able to detoxify the molecule rapidly.

I must briefly explain why endotoxin is so devastating. It can cause direct cell injury with inhibition of gluconeogenesis and protein synthesis, disruption of mitochondria and release of lysosomal enzymes. It activates the complement system and also the kinin system. Its vasoconstrictor potential is very great and in this it is aided by the release of catecholamines, sympathetic nervous system activation and stimulation of the renin-angiotensin mechanism. Finally it causes intravasular coagulation. The microthrombosis may be permanent because it destroys vascular endothelium, so removing the local fibrinolytic potential, additionally it. inhibits the reticulo-endothelial clearance capacity for fibrin and activated coagulation products.

Endotoxinaemia in patients with septic shock or superimposed on traumatic shock has been shown to account for 'shock lung', otherwise known as the adult respiratory distress syndrome. Since endotoxin may occur in drinking water and milk, it has been suggested that its absorption from the permeable gut of the neonate accounts for some cases of 'cot death'. Certainly in infantile gastroenteritis endotoxin is absorbed and accounts for the high mortality that can occur. In adults it also accounts for many cases of acute kidney failure. We have come to the realization that many acute renal failure patients have a Shwartzman reaction, from the detailed studies of intravascular coagulation that we have done at the time of onset of acute renal failure. The Shwartzman reaction, may I remind you, is the production of renal cortical necrosis in the rabbit by two spaced doses of endotoxin given approximately 18 hours apart. We now know that a continuous infusion of smaller doses has a similar effect. Shwartzman described his reaction in 1929, its relevance to the kidney was emphasized by Apitz and by Sanarelli in 1935, and, although there have been many pointers to its relevance tc human disease coming mainly from the French and German schools of medicine, it has been only recently, with the introduction of the Limulus test for endotoxin, that endotoxinaemia has been directly demonstrated in the plasma of patients at the onset of acute renal failure. (Wardle, 1975a, b). Using the Limulus test the relevance of endotoxin to liver disease has also been emphasized.

The white cells of Limulus polyphemus, a warm water crab, contain a protein which forms a gel when it comes into contact with endotoxin. An assay, of striking sensitivity, which is able to detect nanogram amounts of endotoxin has thus been developed. (Reinhold and Fine, 1971).

Now since the work of Jacob Fine in 1960 (Ravin et al., 1960) it has been known that certainly in some species, the rabbit for example, endotoxinaemia can arise from the bowel flora when the animal is in shock and has an under-perfused bowel. Indeed germ-free animals may be quite resistant to haemorrhagic shock but when coliform organisms are put into the bowel beforehand, then the shock is lethal. (Witznitzer et al., 1960). An animal's reaction to shock depends on the nature of its bowel flora, the type of E. Coli antibodies that it has and its degree of endotoxin tolerance. The Limulus assay has shown that man also can absorb endotoxin from the colon during shock. (Woodruff et al., 1973). It appears that ischaemia of the colonic wall due to vasoconstriction leads to a break-down of the antibacterial defense mechanisms (Fine, 1956). The dog is recognized to develop haemorrhagic or pseudomembranous entero-colitis in shock and equivalent histological effects have been noted in man.

Since Kupffer cells of the liver detoxify endotoxin, and their enhanced peroxidase activity suggests that they may use a free radical attack for destroying whole bacteria, it would be logical to expect more conspicuous effects of endotoxin or septicaemia in patients with liver disease. Patients with cirrhosis have high E. coli antibody titres but nevertheless endotoxinaemia has also been found. Moreover in cirrhosis antigen-antibody complexes can enter the general circulation because of shunts around the damaged liver and inactivity of the Kupffer cells. This is referred to as 'spill-over'. It will account for the intravascular coagulation of cirrhosis. Patients with obstructive jaundice and those with hepatic coma can show endotoxinaemia and intravascular coagulation: they often develop shock lung or kidney failure (Wardle, 1974). In animal experiments transient stasis of blood flow in the portal vein has been shown to result in endotoxinaemia, and, there are in the circulation other RES depressing substances (Gans, 1974; Olcay et al., 1974).

Now we need therefore to be clear about the endotoxin inactivating mechanisms, and how it is that endotoxin can cross the bowel mucosa. Absorption is very rapid. Shreeve and Thomlinson (1972) have shown that in the neonatal pig and the guinea pig, anaphyllactic shock can develop within 5 minutes of putting endotoxin into the bowel and the antigen appears rapidly in the spleen. Hypersensitivity effects must be considered but lack of antibodies to lipid A is striking.

Although antibodies to the closely associated R and O-antigen of endotoxins do contribute to immunity against Gram-negative bacterial infections, their role in endotoxin immunity appears to be minimal. (Watson, 1971). Certainly endotoxin-antibody complexes will be cleared by the RES: such complexes may contribute to hypersensitivity and shock. Endotoxin inactivation in the tolerant animal occurs in the reticulo-endothelial system and is a lysosomal function.

It is thought that when endotoxin enters the circulation it initially becomes bound to an alpha-1-lipoprotein and that final inactivation is accomplished by means of an alpha-l-globulin, which is heat labile. Both proteins have non-specific esterase activity and they function efficiently when the plasma ionic calcium is low (Skarnes, 1970). In fact a low plasma calcium does occur in endotoxinaemia. Although complement is activated by endotoxin, complement does not appear to contribute to endotoxin inactivation. Indeed heating serum to 55 °C for 30 minutes does not prevent endotoxin inactivation.

Freter (1974) has recently reviewed the defence mechanisms against gut bacteria. In the first place there is competition between the bacterial species in a healthy bowel, and secondly local copro-immunoglobulin prevents adhesion of bacteria to the mucosal cells. Thirdly in the immune animal IgG and IgM immunoglobulins of the serum permeate the bowel wall and exert a bactericidal effect at the mucosa. It should be stressed that local antibacterial immunity acts synergistically with bacterial antagonisms. Moreover it is to be noted that although parenteral administration of formalinized bacteria produces systemic and local gut antibody, that this does not always prevent colonization with E. coli serotypes. (Kenny et al., 1974).

So I have to end by speculating on the factors which allow endotoxin into the body. We are certain that stasis in the splanchnic capillary bed as a result of shock or the stasis of portal hypertension plays a role. This may interfere with local immunity. In some species the bowel mucosa may ulcerate as a result of intense vasoconstriction. The endotoxin may not enter the blood stream directly but enter first through the bowel serosa into the peritoneal cavity, lymphatic absorption is involved. The important problem is to explain what happens at the level of the mucosal cells: it could be that impairment of energy production allows endotoxin to slip between cells or that mucosal lysosomal mechanisms are ineffectual or actually aid endotoxin passage.

Alternatively it could be that only motile bacteria can cross the intestinal mucosa. Whichever way it is I hope that I have indicated that there is much scope for research on this vital topic.

References

Fine, J. (1956). Effect of peripheral vascular collapse on the antibacterial defense mechanisms. Ann. N.Y. Acad. Sci., **66**, 329

Freter, R. (1974). Interactions between mechanisms controlling the intestinal flora. Am. J. Clin. Nutr., **27**, 1409

Gans, H. (1974). Effect of ligation of the heptic artery or occlusion of the portal vein on the development of endotoxinaemia. Surg. Gynecol. Obstet., **139**, 689

Kenny, J.F., Weinert, D. W. and Gray, J. A. (1974). Failure of specific immunity to alter intestinal colonization of infants and adults. J. Infect. Dis., 129, 10

Olcay, I., Kitahama, A., Miller, R. H., Drapanas, T., Trejo, R. A. and DiLuzio, N. R. (1974). Reticulo-endothelial dysfunction and endo-toxinaemia following portal vein occlusion. Surgery, **75**, 64

Ravin, H. A., Rowley, D., Jenkins, C. F. and Fine, J. (1960). On the absorption of bacterial endotoxin from the gastrointestinal tract of the normal and shocked animal. Journal of Experimental Medicine, **112**, 783

Reinhold, R. B. and Fine, J. (1971). A technique for quantitative measurement of endotoxin in human plasma. Proc. Soc. Exp. Biol. Med., **137**, 334

Shreeve, B. J. and Thomlinson, J. R. (1972). Absorption of E. coli endotoxin by the neonatal pig. J. Md. Microbiol., **5**, 55

Skarnes, R. C. (1970). Host defence against bacterial endotoxinaemia. J. Exp. Med., 132, 300

Watson, D. W. (1971). Gram negative sepsis. Beechams Pharmaceuticals Symposium. Publisher R. E. Fuiz. Clifton, N. J. 07012. Ed. J. P. Sandford. p.40-46

Wardle, E. N. (1974). Fibrinogen catabolism and endotoxinaemia in liver disease. Arch. Surg. 109, 741

Wardle, E. N. (1975a). Endotoxin and acute renal failure. Nephron, **14**, 321

Wardle, E. N. (1975b). Endotoxinaemia and the pathogenesis of acute renal failure. Q. J. Med., **44**, 389

Witznitzer, T., Schweinburg, F. B., Atkin, N. and Fine, J. (1960). On the relation of the size of the intra-intestinal pool of endotoxin to the development of irreversibility in hemorrhagic shock. J. Exp. Med., **112**, 1167

Woodruff, P. W. H., Carroll, D., Koizumi, S. and Fine, J. (1973). Role of the intestinal flora in major trauma. J. Infect. Dis., Suppl. 128, s.290

POSTSCRIPT

(1) Our own studies of Kupffer cell clearances in relation to liver blood flow in man have in fact shown that Kupffer cells are actively phagocytosing in liver disease and that there is Kupffer cell hyperplasia. Thus failure to clear endotoxin or food antigens can only be due to shunting.

(ii) It is now certain that most healthy persons have very low anti-lipid A antibodies. Raised titres are found in patients with inflammatory bowel disease.

Marget, W., Schüssler, P., Kruis, W., Weinzierl, M., Rindfleishch, G. (1976). A study of lipid-A antibody titres in Crohn's disease, ulcerative colitis and acute enteritis. Infection, **4**, 110

(iii) More is known about the role of O-antigens in relation to immunity.

e.g. McLean, A. J. (1977). Relation between E. coli endotoxicity and the immunisation status of normal adult guinea pigs. Br. J. Exp. Pathol., **58**, 255

(iv) Nolan has studied endotoxin absorption through bowel mucosa and claims that Michaelis Menten kinetics are followed.

Nolan, J. P., Hare, D. K., McDevitt, J. J., Ali, M. V. (1977). In vitro studies of intestinal endotoxin absorption. Gastroenterology, **72**, 434

19

Antibody-facilitated digestion and the consequences of its failure

F. H. Y. GREEN and D. L. J. FREED

Immunological and digestive mechanisms are alike in that they break down protein and saccharide macromolecules into smaller units, which are thereby rendered both harmless and usable. Metchnikoff considered immunity to be one aspect of digestion and indeed in primitive animals both functions are served by one mechanism — phagocytosis.

Many common dietary macromolecules (especially proteins) are antigenic (Truelove and Jewell, 1975) and elicit local immune responses (Wansbrough-Jones et al., 1975), and it has been suggested that the local antibody produced interferes with their absorption by forming an impermeable barrier in the glycocalyx (Walker et al., 1975). Yet nearly 100% of ingested protein is absorbed rapidly and efficiently from the gut lumen (Wiseman, 1964), much of it directly into the enterocyte as oligopeptide (Silk, 1974). In this form it is still likely to be antigenic as 3-6 amino acids is the optimal size for antigenic determinants (Kabat, 1968). There thus appears to be a contradiction.

Initial digestion of dietary proteins occurs in the gut lumen under the influence of gastric and pancreatic enzymes, but complete breakdown into amino acids would require exposure to the enzymes for about 200 hours (Fisher, 1954) and therefore many (possibly most) proteins reach the intestinal mucosa in the form of oligopeptides. Some of these are hydrolysed within the brush border or at the cell membrane (Matthews, 1974; Ugolev, 1972) and others are taken up intact by the enterocyte, with intracellular hydrolysis (Silk, 1974; Matthews, 1974). The uptake mechanism for oligopeptides is more efficient than that responsible for amino acids (Silk, 1974), and a number of observations would suggest that they are absorbed by different pathways. For example, patients with Hartnup disease and cystinuria, who cannot absorb mixtures of free amino acids, can utilize them if they are presented in the form of peptides (Silk, 1974; Matthews, 1974). Both uptake mechanisms are active, continuing in the face of an increasing concentration gradient and requiring the expenditure of energy, and it has been inferred from a number of experimental data that specific receptors exist at the enterocyte surface. There are about 400 dipeptides, 6000 tripeptides and so on, so the diversity of receptors required for all possible oligopeptides is considerable.

We suggest that antibodies are admirably suited to function as the proposed cell surface receptors, and that the processing of peptide-antibody complex by the enterocyte is analogous to the function served, in the systemic context, by the body phagocytes. Antigenic proteins are thus absorbed by a process of opsonization.

Intestinal antibodies exist in the form of secretory IgA (SIgA), with a smaller amount of SIgM. SIgA consists of two IgA sub-units linked by J chain and coupled to secretory component, the latter being a glycoprotein produced by epithelial cells. The protective function of secretory antibodies has been well documented (Walker and Hong, 1973; Hill and Porter, 1974; Williams and Gibbons, 1972), and specific secretory antibody levels correspond well with resistance to reinfection by pathogenic organisms (Waldman and Ganguly, 1974). Immuno-fluorescence studies (Brandtzaeg, 1974) show that SIgA is prominent within the apical cytoplasm and brush border of the crypt epithelial cells, with progressive diminution as the enterocyte ascends the villus. Secretory component (SC) is located within the apical cytoplasm, Golgi region and along the plasma membrane of the same cells. From these 'static' data has evolved the accepted theory of SIgA production (Brandtzaeg, 1974), which states that dimeric IgA molecules, liberated from the local plasma cells, are linked to SC at the enterocyte membrane, and then transported into and through it, to be exported via its luminal border.

This model does not, however, explain the immunofluorescence findings at other mucosal sites, exposed to the external environment but **not** concerned with the absorption of food. In the gall bladder (Chen and Tobe, 1974; Green and Fox, 1972) and female genital tract (Rebello et al., 1975) the SIgA is confined to the basement membrane region, interepithelial spaces and the mucosal brush border; intraepithelial IgA is scanty or absent. Even in the chronically inflamed gall bladder, where large numbers of subepithelial plasma cells are seen, no intraepithelial IgA is seen except (significantly) for areas showing intestinal metaplasia (Green and Fox, 1972). It seems necessary to conclude that where only a 'protective' function is required the transepithelial route is not needed; that IgA passes via the intercellular spaces onto the surface when the tight junctions are opened under the influence of vasoactive inflammatory agents (Murray et al., 1971). Nor is the transepithelial

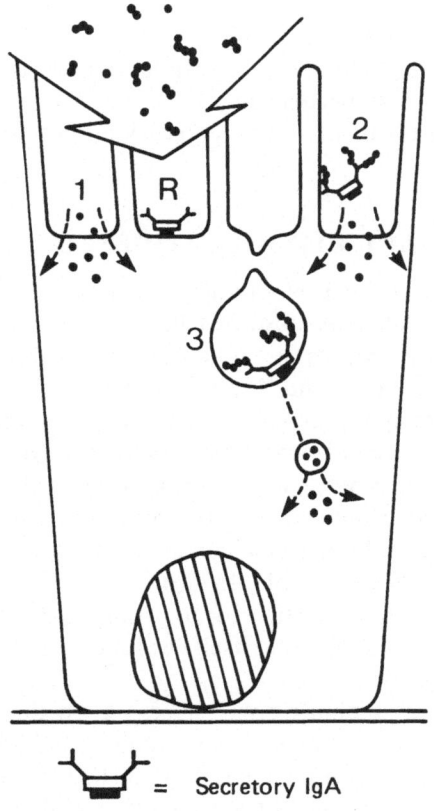

= Secretory IgA

Figure 1 Proposed pathways for protein absorption into the enterocyte. (1) Amino acids from luminal hydrolysis are taken up by a specific pathway. Oligopeptides bind to antibody-receptor (R) and are either (2) degraded by brush-border proteases, or (3) taken into vacuoles for intracellular hydrolysis

route needed for the linkage of IgA to SC, since this will happen spontaneously in vitro (Mach, 1970). It is only used when an additional function is required of the antibodies.

Our model (Figure 1) envisages that IgA is taken up by the undifferentiated cells in the crypt. This store of SIgA is used up in keeping the enterocyte brush border richly supplied with protein-binding receptors, which serve to hold the protein substrates firmly in contact with the appropriate enzymes. Sequential degradation of protein occurs within the brush border. Peptides penetrating to the cell membrane are bound by membrane-associated antibody, endocytosed and hydrolysed within the cell.

The model has advantages:

1. It accounts for the two important functions of the gastro-intestinal tract with one mechanism.

2. It suggests ways in which the enterocyte may protect itself from dietary poisons.

EXPERIMENTAL AND CLINICAL EVIDENCE

The hypothesis is supported by a number of data:

1. Ferritin molecules are absorbed into the hamster enterocyte by micropinocytosis; this process is enhanced by previous immunization with the antigen (Bockman and Winborn, 1966).

1. Intraperitoneally immunized rats show increased binding, immunologically specific, of bovine serum albumin (BSA) to antibodies in the enterocyte glycocalyx, with increased proteolysis and reduced passage of undegraded antigen to the serosal side of the small bowel (Walker et al., 1975a). This increased breakdown requires the presence of pancreatic enzymes (Walker et al., 1975b).

3. Secretory antibody can form complexes with proteases (Counitchansky et al., 1970) being itself resistant to proteolysis (Tomasi and Bienenstock, 1968).

4. Protein-calorie malnutrition causes a syndrome of severe infections with diarrhoea. Three recent studies (Sirisinha et al., 1974; Chandra, 1975; Heyworth and Green, unpublished) have shown that the illness is associated with poor SIgA production, and that this does not return to normal even after full clinical recovery. This suggests that the illness is not an inexorable consequence of poor diet, but that in a critical nutritional environment the efficiency of the secretory antibody mechanism determines the outcome.

5. Six out of fourteen patients suffering from severe post-vagotomy diarrhoea were shown (McLoughlin et al., 1976) to have deficiency of IgA, IgM and IgE. The authors reason that the extra stress of vagotomy may unmask an occult antibody defect.

6. Immunodeficient patients lacking intestinal antibodies frequently suffer from diarrhoea and malabsorption, and also from microbial colonization of the small bowel. Conventionally the chain of causation has been pictured thus:—

(i) IMMUNE DEFICIT $\rightarrow$ MICROBIAL COLONIZATION $\rightarrow$ DIARRHOEA

but it is also possible to sketch at least three other pathways, thus:—

(ii) IMMUNE DEFICIT $\rightarrow$ INEFFICIENT DIGESTION (MALABSORPTION)

(iii) IMMUNE DEFICIT $\rightarrow$ INEFFICIENT DIGESTION $\rightarrow$ MEDIUM SUITABLE FOR MICROBIAL PROLIFERATION

(iv) SMALL AMOUNT Ab $\rightarrow$ ANTIGEN EXCESS $\rightarrow$ SOLUBLE IMMUNE COMPLEX FORMATION
+
NORMAL AMOUNT Ag

$\rightarrow$ TYPE 3 HYPERSENSITIVITY $\rightarrow$ DIARRHEOA + MALABSORPTION

The intestinal symptoms often respond to prolonged courses of antibiotics, particularly metronidazole. These cases would favour (i) or (iv) since imidazole drugs have anti-inflammatory/immunoactive properties as well as microbicidal capability (Taylor, 1966; Sewell, 1976).

CLINICAL IMPLICATIONS

Coeliac disease (gluten-sensitive enteropathy)

Two essentially different mechanisms have been proposed to account for the mucosal lesion in coeliac disease:—
(i) defective digestion of a toxic factor in gluten, and
(ii) allergy to gluten.

We propose that coeliac disease results from a defect of antibody-facilitated digestion, in which the antibodies normally responsible for the utilization/detoxication of gluten are produced either in small quantity or poor quality (avidity). Either would result in soluble immune complex formation. Soluble complex is relatively unappetizing to phagocytic cells, and therefore would not be readily endocytosed by the enterocyte. Instead complement would be fixed, causing local inflammation (Type 3 hypersensitivity). There is abundant evidence of soluble-complex deposition in the coeliac mucosa with the fixation of complement (Lancet, 1974; Shiner and Ballard, 1972). Disease results, we suggest, both from the direct toxicity of gluten (Hudson et al., 1976; Weiser and Douglas, 1976) and indirectly via hypersensitivity. This model happily marries the two main theories of gluten toxicity.

The adequacy of specific immune responsiveness is probably controlled (in part) by immune-response (Ir) genes, which are closely connected to the major histocompatibility loci. It is significant in this context that coeliac disease is HLA-associated (Lancet, 1974).

Feeding of human infants

Human breast milk contains antibodies against antigens ingested by the mother (Lancet, 1976), thus providing the infant with passive immunity and at the same time, we suggest, helping the infant digest and absorb its food. Breast milk also contains traces of antigen (including many drugs) derived from the mother's gut (Vorherr, 1974). The resulting complexes are likely to provide active immunization in a non-inflammatory form (cf toxoid-antitoxin floccules for the immunoprophylaxis of diphtheria), thus preparing the child for its subsequent introduction to antigenic food.

Therapeutic implication

If, as we suggest, human breast milk provides both immunity and 'digestivity' in passive and active form, it should be valuable in the treatment of the bowel disorders we have mentioned in this article, viz, coeliac disease (including cases not responding to gluten withdrawal), protein calorie malnutrition, the malabsorption associated with immunodeficiency and post-vagotomy diarrhoea.

References

Bockman, D. E. and Winborn, W. B. (1966). Light and electron microscopy of intestinal ferritin absorption. Observations in sensitized and non-sensitized hamsters (Mesocricetus auratus). Anat. Rec., 155, 603

Brandtzaeg, P. (1974). Mucosal and glandular distribution of immunoglobulin components: differential localization of free and bound secretory component in secretory epithelial cells. J. Immunol., 112, 1553

Chandra, R. K. (1975). Reduced secretory antibody response to live attenuated measles and poliovirus vaccines in malnourished children. Br. Med. J., 2, 583

Chen, S. T. and Tobe, T. (1974). Cellular sites of immunoglobulins V: an immunological study of the human gall-bladder. Digestion, 10, 184

Counitchansky, Y., Berthellier, G. and Got, R. (1970). Mise en evidence et caracterisation des complexes formes entre les immunoglobulines A (IgA) du colostrum humain et la trypsine ou la chymotrypsine. Clin. Chim. Acta, 30, 83

Fisher, R. B. (1954). Protein Metabolism, London: Methuen

Green, F. H. Y. and Fox, H. (1972). An immunofluorescence study of the distribution of immunoglobulin-containing cells in the normal and the inflamed human gall-bladder. Gut, 13, 379

Heyworth, B. and Green, F. H. Y. Unpublished data.

Hill, I. R. and Porter, P. (1974). Studies of bactericidal activity to Escherichia coli of porcine serum and colostral immunoglobulins and the role of lysozyme with secretory IgA. Immunology, 26, 1239

Hudsen, D. A., Cornell, H. J., Purdham, D. R., Rolles, C. H. (1976). Nonspecific cytotoxicity of wheat gliadin components towards cultured human cells. Lancet, i, 339

Kabat, E. A. (1968). Structural concepts in immunology and immunochemistry. (New York: Holt Rinehart & Winston Inc.)

Lancet (1974). The coeliac philosophy. Lancet, ii, 501

Lancet (1976). Oral immunization and antibodies in milk. Lancet, i, 77

Mach, J.-P. (1970). In-vitro combination of human and bovine free secretory component with IgA of various species. Nature, 228, 1278

McLoughlin, G. A., Bradley, J., Chapman, D. M., Temple, J. G., Hede, J. E. and McFarland, J. (1976). IgA deficiency and severe post-vagotomy diarrhoea. Lancet, i, 168

Matthews, D. M. (1974). Absorption of amino acids and peptides from the intestine. Clin. Endocrinol. Metab., 3, 3

Murray, M., Jarrett, W. F. H. and Jennings, F. W. (1971). Mast cells and macromolecular leak in intestinal immunological reactions; the influence of sex of rats infected with Nippostrongylus brasiliensis. Immunology, **21**, 17

Rebello, R., Green, F. H. Y. and Fox, H. (1975). A study of the secretory immune system of the female genital tract. Br. J. Obset. Gynaecol., **82**, 812

Sewell, J. R. (1976). Levamisole for rheumatoid arthritis. Lancet, **i**, 651

Shiner, M. and Ballard, J. (1972). Antigen-antibody reactions in jejunal mucosa in childhood coeliac disease after gluten challenge. Lancet, **i**, 1202

Silk, D. B. A. (1974). Progress report: peptide absorption in man. Gut, **15**, 494

Sirisinha, S., Suskind, R., Edelman, R., Asvapaka, C. and Olson, R. E. (1974). Secretory and serum IgA in children with protein-calorie malnutrition. Adv. Exp. Med. Biol., **45**, 389

Taylor, J. A. T. (1966). Pharmacodynamic observations in metronidazole therapy: side effects in endocrine, metabolic and autoimmune disorders. Proc. West. Pharmac. Soc., **9**, 37

Tomasi, T. B. and Bienenstock, J. (1968). Secretory immunoglobulins. Adv. Immunol., **9**, 1

Truelove, S. C. and Jewell, D. P. (1975). The Intestine in allergic disease. In Clinical Aspects of Immunology, P. G. H. Gell, R. R. A. Coombs and P. J. Lachmann, eds. Blackwell. (Oxford: Blackwell Scientific Publications).

Ugolev, A. M. (1972). Progress report: membrane digestion. Gut, **13**, 735-747.

Vorherr, H. (1974). Drug excretion in breast milk. Postgrad. Med., **56**, 97

Waldman, R. H. and Ganguly, R. (1974). The role of the secretory immune system in protection against agents which infect the respiratory tract. Adv. Exp. Med. Biol., **45**, 283

Walker, W. A. and Hong, R. (1973). Immunology of the gastrointestinal tract. J. Pediat., **83**, 517

Walker, W. A., Wu, M., Isselbacher, K. J. and Bloch, K. J. (1975a). Intestinal uptake of macromolecules II. Gastroenterology, **69**, 1223

Walker, W. A., Wu, M., Isselbacher, K. J. and Bloch, K. J. (1975b). Intestinal uptake of macromolecules III. J. Immunol., **115**, 854

Wansbrough-Jones, M. H., Pepys, M. B. and Doe, W. F. (1975).

Antigen-binding cells in rabbits in response to intestinal immunization. Meeting of Brit. Soc. Immunol, 16th Oct., 1975

Weiser, M. M. and Douglas, A. P. (1976). An alternative mechanism for gluten toxicity in coeliac disease. Lancet, i, 567

Williams, R. C. and Gibbons, R. J. (1972). Inhibition of bacterial adherence by secretory IgA: a mechanism of antigen disposal. Science, 177, 697

Wiseman, G. (1964). Absorption from the Small Intestine. (New York and London: Academic Press)

20

Endopeptidase activity of the small intestine

J. F. WOODLEY and E. E. STERCHI

INTRODUCTION

The absorption of antigens intact by the small intestine of mammalian species, presupposes that such antigens are able to survive the digestive capacity of that organ. In this paper, we present evidence to suggest that the enzymic capability of the small intestine, in particular of the brush border membrane, to hydrolyse proteins is high.

METHODS AND RESULTS

It is well known that the mammalian pancreas secretes fluid into the intestinal lumen via the pancreatic duct. This fluid contains the proteolytic enzymes trypsin, chymotrypsin, carboxypeptidases A and B, as well as the rather specific enzyme, elastase. Between them these enzymes have considerable hydrolytic potential of quite wide specificity. All the enzymes are secreted as inactive precursors or proenzymes, and the initial step in the activation is the specific function of the enzyme enterokinase. Enterokinase has been shown to be located in the brush border of the enterocytes of the proximal part of the small intestine (Schmitz et al., 1974) and activation of the proenzymes may therefore take place at or on the brush border membrane. It might be inferred that binding of these proenzymes to the brush border is a prerequisite to activation. Our experimental studies with rats strongly support the view that pancreatic proteolytic enzymes bind to the cell surface or brush border of the epithelial cells.

A crude brush border preparation was prepared from the small intestine of rats. The animals were starved overnight, sacrificed, and the entire small intestine washed with warm (37 °C) physiological saline in situ. The small intestine was removed, everted, and washed further in saline. The mucosa was gently scraped from the intestine and homogenized in 0.33 M sucrose using a high speed blender (Ultra-Turrax, by Janke and Kunkel K.G., Staffen.) The homogenate was centrifuged at 14 000 g for 25 min, and the pellet discarded. The crude brush borders were then collected as a 150 000 g × 60 min pellet.

The proteolytic enzyme activity (endopeptidase) was measured in this crude brush border fraction, by the release of trichloroacetic acid soluble radioactivity, using iodine-125 labelled B chain of insulin as substrate (Wong-Leung and Kenny, 1968). Pancreatic protease activity was measured by assaying with iodine-125 B chain of insulin in the presence of 10^{-3}M diisopropylphosphofluoridate (DFP). This compound is a powerful irreversible inhibitor of serine proteases and as such will inhibit all the pancreatic proteolytic enzymes. At a concentration of 10^{-3}M DFP, 85-90% of the brush border endopeptidase activity was inhibited. These results suggested that most of the endopeptidase activity of the rat brush borders, could be attributed to bound pancreatic enzymes. To confirm this observation, a number of experiments were carried out, in which the flow of pancreatic enzymes into the gut was surgically excluded.

The pancreatic ducts of a number of animals were ligated close to the entrance into the duodenum and the animals allowed to recover. 5-7 days after operation, the animals were sacrificed. The small intestine was washed through with physiological saline and the washings retained for analysis. The mucosa was scraped from the gut and homogenized and fractioned as before. Unoperated litter mates were treated in the same fashion, and used as controls.

Analysis of the gut content washings for peptidase activity using iodine-125 labelled B chain of insulin showed that on average, the endopeptidase of the gut contents was reduced in the experimental to 3% of that of controls, thus confirming the success of the surgical exclusion of pancreatic enzymes. The non-peptidase pancreatic enzyme, amylase, showed a similar reduction. The brush borders prepared from the surgically treated animals and the controls were assayed for peptidase activity in the presence of increasing concentrations of DFP. The results

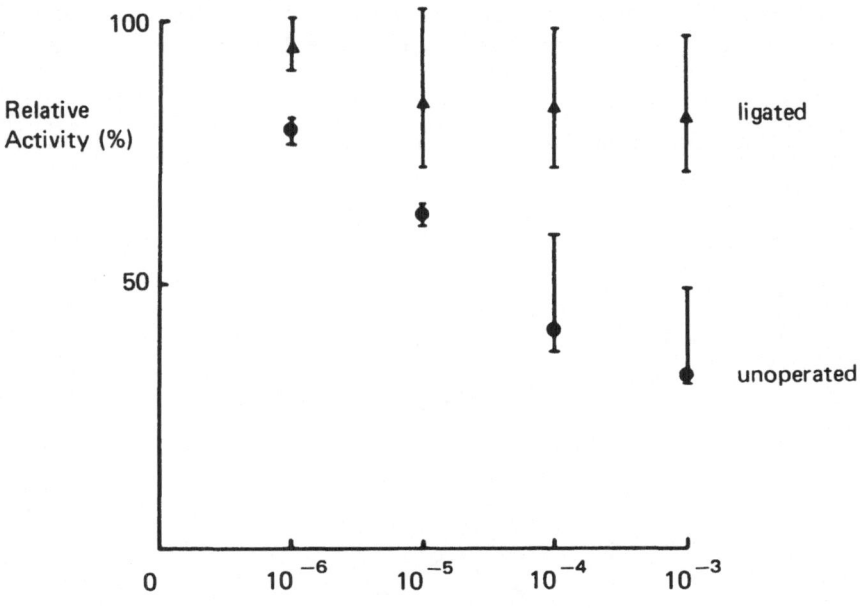

Figure 1 Effect of DFP on endopeptidase activity of crude brush borders prepared from operated and control animals. Each point represents the mean of three animals

are shown in Figure 1, and show that the exclusion of pancreatic juice has removed essentially all the DFP inhibitable endopeptidase activity from the brush border preparation. The total endopeptidase activity was reduced by 55% by the ligation procedure.

These experiments confirmed that most of the endopeptidase activity of crude brush borders from rat, was attributable to pancreatic contamination, and that the enzymes were bound firmly enough to survive repeated washings, and the preparative procedure. The remaining endopeptidase activity, which was uninhibited by DFP, was subsequently shown to be an intrinsic zinc requiring endopeptidase (Woodley, 1969).

In addition to these studies of endopeptidase activity of rat brush borders, we have carried out extensive studies on the peptidase activities of human brush border membranes, using a highly purified membrane preparation.

Purified brush borders were prepared from sections of human small intestine obtained at surgery. The tissue sections were frozen immediately and stored at —20 °C. until required. Figure 2 shows the preparation

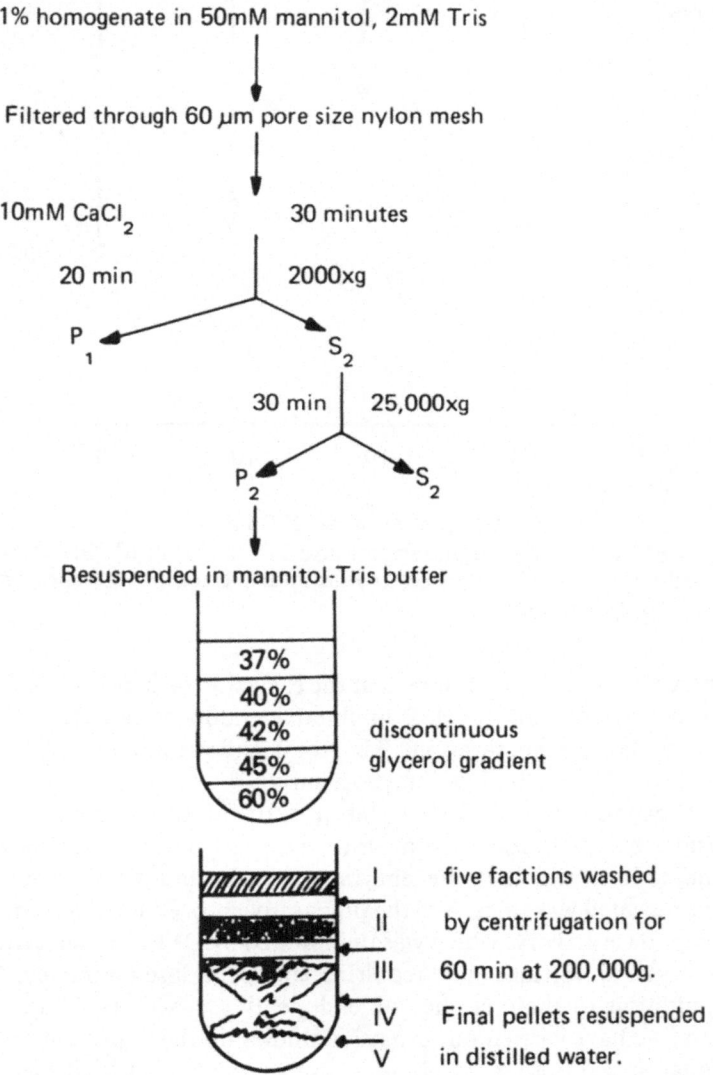

1% homogenate in 50mM mannitol, 2mM Tris

Filtered through 60 μm pore size nylon mesh

10mM CaCl$_2$ 30 minutes

20 min   2000xg

P$_1$ S$_2$

30 min | 25,000xg

P$_2$ S$_2$

Resuspended in mannitol-Tris buffer

37%
40%
42%   discontinuous
45%   glycerol gradient
60%

I   five factions washed
II   by centrifugation for
III   60 min at 200,000g.
IV   Final pellets resuspended
V   in distilled water.

Figure 2 Schematic representation of the purification procedure of human brush border membranes

method, which is a modification of that of Schmitz et al. (1973). The brush borders were obtained in a high state of purity, showing a 50-fold increase in specific activity of the brush border marker enzyme α-glucosidase, and were free from contamination with marker enzymes from other subcellular organelle. This is important when studying brush border peptidases in detail, to be certain that, as there are peptidases in both the lysosomes and cytosol, the activities being studied are genuine brush border enzymes and not contamination. The purified brush border membranes have been tested for peptidase activity with a number of peptidase substrates. With natural peptidases, activity was assayed by measuring the release of free amino acids, which were estimated using L-amino acid oxidase (Donlon and Fottrell, 1971). Activity was also measured using amino acid and peptide naphthylamides. Hydrolysis of these synthetic substrates was followed by fluorimetrically measuring the release of β-naphthylamine (Peters et al., 1975). Iodine-125 labelled B chain of insulin was also used as a substrate.

Table 1 shows a table of results of peptidase activities in purified brush border membranes, as increases in specific activity compared with the homogenate, and as the percentage of activity recovered in the fraction, again compared with the homogenate. A comparison of the increase in specific activity and percentage distribution of a peptidase activity with

Table 1 Peptide activities in brush border

Substrate	Increase in Sp. Act. (Hom = 1)	% Total (Hom = 100)
leu-gly	8.8	2.4
leu-gly-gly	16.5	4.6
phe-gly	17.3	4.8
α-glu- β-naphthylamide	18.6	5.1
leu-leu-leu	22.0	6.1
leu-leu	23.0	6.5
phe-gly-gly	23.4	6.4
tyr-tyr	24.1	6.7
tyr-tyr-tyr	27.9	7.7
tyr-gly	28.5	7.9
tyr-gly-gly	33.8	9.3
Iodine-125 insulin B chain	33.6	9.2
gly-pro- β-naphthylamide	43.8	6.0
α-glucoside	54.0	6.9

the brush border marker enzyme α-glucosidase, indicates whether the peptidase are exclusively located in the brush border membrane, or have a dual location in the brush border and other parts of the cell, particularly the cytoplasm.

It is clear from Table 1 that the brush border membranes are capable of splitting all the substrates tested. However with a number of the substrates tested, notably tyr-tyr-tyr, tyr-gly, tyr-gly-gly, B chain of insulin and gly-pro-β-naphthylamide, the figures on the increase in specific activity and percent recovery, indicate that these activities are predominantly located in the brush border. The latter two activities may be considered as endopeptidase activities, although in the case of the activity against gly-pro-β-naphthylamide, the enzyme is dipeptidyl aminopeptidase IV, which required proline or alanine residues adjacent to the N-terminal amino acid. The enzyme has also been shown to have endopeptidase activity but the specificity for proline residues is maintained (Kenny et al., 1976). The activities against the tripeptides have been clearly shown by thin layer chromatography to be aminopeptidase activities.

CONCLUSIONS

From the data presented it can be seen that the brush border membrane offers a formidable barrier to the passage of intact proteins. Evidence from the study with rats shows that pancreatic enzymes can bind to the surface of the enterocytes. This evidence, coupled with the fact the enzyme which activates the pancreatic proteases, enterokinase, is located in the brush border membrane, suggests that the cell surface of the enterocyte is a major site for the hydrolysis of proteins by pancreatic endopeptidases. In addition to the bound pancreatic peptidases, the studies with purified human brush border membranes, show that the membranes contain activity against a wide range of substrates. Clearly the data indicate that the aminopeptidase of the enterocyte against tripeptides, and the endopeptidase activity against B chain of insulin and gly-pro-β-naphthylamide are predominantly located in the brush border membrane.

For a protein molecule such as an antibody to be absorbed intact by the small intestine, it must have properties which will prevent it from being hydrolysed by pancreatic and intrinsic brush border peptidases.

ACKNOWLEDGEMENTS

We wish to acknowledge the Wellcome Trust and the Erziehungs-direktion des Kantons Bern, Switzerland, for financial support.

References

Donlon, J. and Fottrell, P. F. (1971). Quantitative determination of intestinal peptide hydrolase activity using L-amino acid oxidase. Clin. Chim. Acta, **33**, 345

Kenny, A. J., Booth, A. G., George, S. G., Ingram, J., Kershaw, D., Wood, E. J. and Young, A. R. (1976). Dipeptidyl peptidase IV, a kidney brush border serine peptidase. Biochem. J., **157**, 169

Peters, T. J., Heath, J. R., Wansbrough-Jones, M. H. and Doe, W. F. (1975). Enzyme activities and properties of lysosomes and brush borders in jejunal biopsies from control subjects and patients with coeliac disease. Clin. Sci. Mol. Med., **48**, 259

Schmitz, J., Preiser, H., Maestracci, D., Ghosh, B. K., Cerda, J. J., and Crane, R. K. (1973). Purification of the human intestinal brush border membrane. Biochim. Biophys. Acta, **323**, 98

Schmitz, J., Prieser, H., Maestracci, D., Crane, R. K., Troesch, V. and Hadorn, B. (1974). Subcellular localisation of enterokinase in human small intestine. Biochim. Biophys. Acta, 343, 435

Wong-Leung, Y. L. and Kenny, A. J. (1968). Some properties of a microsomal peptidase in rat kidney. Biochem. J., **110**, 5P

Woodley, J. F. (1969). Studies on peptidases in the intestinal mucosa and other tissues of the rat. Thesis, University of Leeds

21

The traffic of lymphocytes through the gut of mammals

J. G. HALL

INTRODUCTION

Although there has been always a strong circumstantial connection between the lymphoreticular system and the processes of immunity it is only in the last two decades that it has become generally accepted that lymphoid cells provide the cellular basis for specific immunological reactions. Similarly, even since the observations of Joseph Conrad Peyer in 1677 it has been known that the gut is supplied abundantly with lymphoid tissue. In the intervening years many strange notions have been advanced to explain this association but it is only recently that coherent ideas have emerged about the role of the gut-associated lymphoid tissue (GALT) in immune reactions.

On general grounds it would seem that the gut is in need of special protection; it has a vast surface area which is adapted especially for absorption and yet it is in direct contact with the external environment and is exposed constantly to its own peculiar microflora as well as to bacteria, viruses and toxins in the diet. It is hardly surprising therefore that throughout recorded history man and his agricultural livestock have been devastated by enteric infections. It was perhaps no accident that Pasteur's first successful active immunization procedure was directed against an enteric infection of domestic fowls. However it was not until 1922 that Davies reported the presence of antibodies to intestinal pathogens in the stools of dysentery patients. Experimental work on guinea pigs (Burrows, Elliott and Havens, 1947) confirmed the existence of 'copro antibody' and by the end of the 1950s there was a substantial body of evidence (reviewed by Pierce, 1959) supporting the concept of specialized 'muco antibodies' which protected mucous surfaces as a sort of 'antiseptic paint'.

At about the same time the idea that lymphocytes were implicated in the genesis of the plasma cells that produced antibodies was becoming established (McMaster, 1961) and a little while later the characteristic immunoglobulin of mucous secretions, IgA, was identified and characterized by Heremans and his colleagues (Heremans, 1974). It soon became clear that the lymphoid tissue beneath mucous membranes and in particular the lamina propria of the gut, was particularly rich in plasma cells that secreted IgA (Tourville et al., 1969). Also these plasma cells could be generated apparently in response to local stimuli such as viruses or bacterial antigens applied to the gut mucosa (Ogra and Karzon, 1969; Porter, Noakes and Allen, 1970) so that specific IgA antibodies were produced locally with little or no corresponding increase in the titre of conventional antibody in the systemic blood circulation. This apparent dissociation between local antibody production at mucous surfaces and the systemic humoral response is something that has to be borne in mind when the traffic of lymphoid cells is being considered.

Quite apart from this direct and practical interest in immunity in the gut, immunobiologists were becoming interested in the subject for more basic and recondite reasons. Between 1955 and 1960 several experimenters showed that the removal of the bursa of Fabricius (a lymphoid organ associated with the cloaca) from neonatal chicks prevented the animals from making significant amounts of immuno-globulins (Miller, 1963). A search for a mammalian 'bursal equivalent' was mounted and has continued without decisive avail to this day but Good and his colleagues have suggested that parts of the mammalian GALT may have a function analogous to that of the avian bursa in the ontogeny of immune reactivity (Cooper and Lawton, 1973).

Finally, the central theme of this book, i.e. the absorption of colostral proteins by the gut of neonatal mammals presents another facet of the interface between gastrointestinal physiology and immunology. Also, it is becoming apparent that even the normal adult bowel can absorb tiny, but immunologically significant, amounts of intact and potentially immunogenic macromolecules and clinicians are becoming concerned increasingly about the role of allergic phenomena in the

208

aetiology of various chronic bowel diseases. Obviously, there is such a vast area for discussion and experiment that one cannot proceed without making a few generalizations. Unfortunately, these are even more dangerous than usual. The transfer of immunoglobulins from mother to offspring, either via the placenta or via the colostrum, may have an important bearing on the development of the GALT but there are very great differences between species in the details of diet, lactation, placentation and the pre-natal development of the GALT which must raise suspicions about definitive statements, however succinct and pithy they may seem at first sight. The following account of lymphocyte traffic through the GALT is not proffered as an exception to this rule.

ANATOMY AND PHYSIOLOGY OF THE GALT

Like most tissues the intestine is provided with lymph nodes; the tissue fluid formed in the interstitial spaces of the intestinal wall drains to and is filtered by the mesenteric lymph nodes, the efferent ducts from which join to form the intestinal lymph duct. The mesenteric nodes are similar in general structure to the other nodes of the body but betray evidence of continual antigenic stimulation so that the intestinal lymph contains always a significant number of large lymphoid blast cells, i.e. immunoblasts (Heath, Lascelles and Morris, 1962; Hall, 1971), together with the usual small lymphocytes which populate the efferent lymph from any lymph node. These small lymphocytes are derived mainly from the blood by extravasation through specialized post capillary venules in the deep cortical regions of the node (Gowans and Knight, 1964).

Although the mesenteric nodes comprise the most obvious part of the GALT there is also a substantial amount of lymphoid tissue in the wall of the gut. Much of this is dispersed apparently randomly in the lamina propria between the basement membrane of the epithelium and the muscular coats and is comprised of small lymphocytes, lymphoid blast cells (immunoblasts) and mature plasma cells. In addition there are microscopic nodules or follicles of closely packed lymphoid tissue that may contain germinal zones. These follicles may aggregate to form macroscopically obvious structures, the Peyer's patches. Such patches are covered by a sheet of columnar-cuboidal epithelium which lacks the villous structure characteristic of the rest of the gut. The Peyer's patches are another major site of the recirculation of small lymphocytes (Gowans and Knight, 1964), i.e. the process whereby small lymphocytes continually extravasate and are then returned to the blood via the lymph

209

stream. Many of these small lymphocytes are thymus derived (T cells) and the micro-anatomical site of their recirculation is in the interfollicular areas between the lymphoid follicles (Parrott, de Sousa and East, 1966; de Sousa, 1973). This recirculation of small lymphocytes through the Peyer's patch gives the peripheral lymph, i.e. lymph in transit in the small lacteals that connect the wall of the gut to the mesenteric nodes, a uniquely high content of small lymphocytes (Hopkins and Hall, unpublished observations). Peripheral lymph from other organs and tissues contains, in health, very few white cells (Smith, McIntosh and Morris, 1970). Peripheral intestinal lymph also contains significant numbers of lymphoid blast cells; presumably these are generated in the lamina propria but some may come also from the Peyer's patches. In addition, intestinal lymph, be it peripheral or post-nodal, contains the chylomicra and any other macromolecular material absorbed from the gut lumen.

In most large mammals macroscopically obvious Peyer's patches are present well before birth and there is good evidence that even in this antigen-free environment the recirculation of small lymphocytes is proceeding vigourously (Pearson, Simpson-Morgan and Morris, 1976). In rodents however the Peyer's patches only appear around the time of birth (Ferguson and Parrott, 1972). Before birth the lamina propria of most mammals is only very sparsely populated and it is not until after a considerable period of post natal growth and development that a full complement of plasma cells is present.

DETAILS OF LYMPHOCYTE TRAFFIC

Mention has been made above of the continual traffic of recirculating lymphocytes which passes through the Peyer's patches and all the lymph nodes of the body. Those who believe in a clonal selection theory of acquired immunity (Burnet, 1959) suggest, not unreasonably, that by this means each unit of organised lymphoid tissue is supplied, continuously, with a vast population of immunologically competent cells from which those with appropriate genetic potential may be selected to react with antigens which have become localized in the phagocytic cells of the node. This idea is attractive and logical but awaits experimental proof.

However, the phenomenon that really focused the attention of cellular immunologists on the gut was the behaviour of the lymph-borne immunoblasts. Gowans and Knight (1964) showed first that the large lymphoid immunoblasts collected in the thoracic duct lymph of rats, and labelled in vitro with radioactive precursors of DNA, 'homed' back quickly to the lamina propria of the small gut after they had been injected intravenously into syngeneic recipients. This was soon confirmed (Griscelli, Vassalli and McCluskey, 1969; Hall and Smith, 1970), and blast cells teased from mesenteric nodes, but not from somatic nodes, were shown to behave in the same way (Guy-Grand, Griscelli and Vassalli, 1974). It was also shown that many of these blasts later became plasma cells (Gowans and Knight, 1964; Hall, Parry and Smith, 1972) and it had been known for some time that, in general, many lymph-borne immunoblasts were antibody forming plasma-blasts (Hall, 1971) and that some of those in rat thoracic lymph were concerned with the production of IgA (Mandel and Asofsky, 1968). However, at first little evidence could be found that this homing of immunoblasts to the gut was mediated by an immunological affinity for dietary or microbial antigens in the lumen of the gut. The phenomenon occurred just as abundantly in antigen free situations such as caesarian-delivered neonatal rats (Halstead and Hall, 1972), fetal sheep in utero (Hopkins and Hall, unpublished observations) and heterotopic transplants of sterile, fetal gut (Moore and Hall, 1972). More recently Pierce and Gowans (1975) have shown that in rats that have been sensitized systemically to cholera toxoid, immunologically specific immunoblasts accumulate preferentially in the lamina of regions of the gut that have been challenged locally with the specific antigen. Evidently, the immunological specificity of the blasts can play some role in guiding them to their destination but this seems, at the moment, to be a secondary effect which is superimposed on a basic 'gut-seeking' property.

At first, I was inclined to believe that immunoblasts generated in any node could home to the gut (Moore and Hall, 1972) but there was evidence against this (Griscelli et al., 1969; Guy-Grand et al., 1974). The question was settled directly by comparing, in unanaesthetized sheep, the in vivo distribution of radio-labelled immunoblasts obtained either from intestinal lymph, or from the efferent lymph of peripheral somatic lymph nodes (PSLNs) (Hopkins and Hall, 1976). This work showed quite unmistakeably that blasts from intestinal lymph homed to the gut; those from PSLNs did not, they went mainly to the spleen. Also, it was shown, in general conformity with Beh and Lascelles (1974), that although lymph-borne immunoblasts contain IgG and IgM the intestinal lymph contains in addition a large proportion of cells that contain IgA.

Clearly, it is tempting to suggest that IgA, or a closely associated molecule, is the receptor on the surface of immunoblasts that endows them with the ability to extravasate in the lamina propria of the small intestine. While this cannot be ruled out there is evidence against it. In the first place, by no means all the intestinal immunoblasts contain IgA and in the second, and more compellingly Sprent has shown recently (1976) that T immunoblasts, from the thoracic duct lymph of mice, also home to the gut, going mainly to the interfollicular regions near Peyer's patches. Almost by definition T cells do not synthesize detectable amounts of Ig and so it is difficult to propose that such molecules play a major role in the homing process. The possibility that some such humoral factor could be adsorbed passively on to the surface of the T cells cannot be excluded but in the absence of positive data it must remain rather remote.

The ultimate fate of the immunoblasts in the gut is uncertain also. Presumably the B, Ig-containing immunoblasts develop into plasma cells which, after a brief life span devoted to the production of antibody, simply die out and make room for the newcomers which are arriving continually. The function of the T immunoblasts is less easy to understand. Probably they offer a trophic, helper function in the generation of local IgA responses which are believed to require the participation of T cells (Guy-Grand et al., 1975). The whole question of the induction of immune responses in the GALT is obscure. Any antigen that actually penetrates the gut wall and is carried to the mesenteric nodes may obviously initiate a response in the usual way (Hall, 1971) but the massive entry of antigen in this way is hardly compatible with health or, indeed, life. Many responses are induced apparently in the wall of the gut as such (Ogra and Karzon, 1969; Porter et al., 1970) and it is believed that Peyer's patches have a special role in the transport, trapping and processing of antigens (Bockman and Cooper, 1973). Nonetheless, even though some of the lymphoid cells in Peyer's patches may be precursors of cells which ultimately turn into IgA producing plasma cells in other sites (Craig and Cebra, 1971), antibody forming cells are found but rarely in the patches themselves (Bienenstock and Dolezel, 1971). Perhaps the rather peculiar and circuitous journey made by the cells of the GALT, first into the lymph and then, via the blood, back to other regions of the GALT, is a necessary experience for the proper development of the cells' potentialities. At the moment, though, we just do not know enough to give a satisfactory explanation of these events.

The large scale homing of immunoblasts from intestinal lymph back to the GALT naturally made us wonder whether the small lymphocytes of the GALT had any similar propensity. To test this, small lymphocytes were collected from either the intestinal or intermediate somatic lymph of unanaesthetized sheep, labelled in vitro with chromium-51, washed and reinfused intravenously (Scollay, Hopkins and Hall, 1976). Somewhat to our surprise we found quite unequivocally in each experiment that cells collected from intestinal lymph reappeared later in that lymph, whereas cells from the efferent lymph of PSLNs reappeared in that compartment. The distinction between somatic and intestinal recirculation was not absolute but was definite enough to be easily demonstrable. The cells used in the experiments were a mixture of T and B cells (Scollay, Hall and Orlans, 1976) but we do not know whether both types are equally capable of recirculating through their native lymphoid tissue.

These findings are all fairly recent and it would be pointless to attempt any real exegesis at this stage. However, what does seem to be emerging

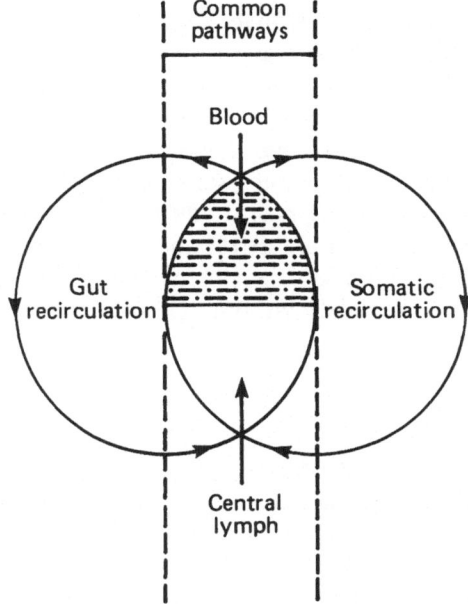

Figure 1 Diagram to show the two principal systems of lymphocyte recirculation. Small lymphocytes recirculate continually from blood to lymph by extravasation in the lymphoid tissue associated with the gut (left) or in the peripheral somatic lymph nodes (right). Immunoblasts, which arise from small lymphocytes that have reacted to antigenic stimuli, leave their parent tissue, recirculate once and home back to their tissue of origin. All cells share a common pathway, first in the central lymph of the major lymphatic trunks and, later, in the blood

fairly clearly is that the circulating lymphocytes of mammals partition between one or other of two major recirculation pathways; the GALT on the one hand, and the somatic and splenic lymphoid tissue on the other. This applies probably to both B and T cells, irrespective of whether they are small lymphocytes or whether they are in the blast phase. However, all types share a final common pathway, first in major lymph trunks such as the thoracic duct and then, briefly, in the blood. (Figure 1.) Unfortunately, it is from one or other of these compartments that clinicians or laboratory workers often collect their starting material. The lymphocytes they collect may be even more heterogeneous than has been recognized hitherto. This dichotomy between the GALT and the somatic/splenic lymphoid tissue can be observed also in the natural history of malignant lymphomata. Hodgkin's disease may involve any of the somatic lymph nodes and the spleen but only rarely involves the mesenteric nodes and gut. Conversely, some of the mesenteric lymphomata common in the Near and Middle East and associated often with alpha-chain disease, may show massive involvement of the GALT co-existing with quite normal peripheral nodes. It is unlikely that these two distinct recirculation pathways have no purpose other than the amusement of biologists and pathologists. There is evidence already that immune responses in the GALT may modify later systemic responses to the original antigen (André et al., 1975) and it seems plausible that this sort of co-operation could do much to ensure the immunological protection of the individual without, at the same time, causing disasterous allergic reactions.

References

André, C., Heremans, J. F., Vaerman, J. P. and Cambiasco, C. L. (1975). A mechanism for the induction of immunological tolerance by antigen feeding: Antigen-antibody complexes. J. Exp. Med., **142,** 1509

Beh, K. J. and Lascelles, A. K. (1974). Class specificity of intracellular and surface immunoglobulin of cells in popliteal and intestinal lymph of sheep. Aust. J. Exp. Biol. Med. Sci., **52,** 505

Bienenstock, J. and Dolezel, J. (1971). Peyer's patches: lack of specific antibody containing cells after oral and parenteral immunization. J. Immunol., **106,** 938

Bockman, D. E. and Cooper, M. D. (1973). Pinocytosis by epithelium associated with lymphoid follicles in the bursa of Fabricius, appendix and Peyer's patches: an electron microscope study. Am. J. Anat., **136**, 455

Burnet, F. M. (1959). The Clonal Selection Theory of Acquired Immunity. p.83. Cambridge University Press

Burrows, W., Elliot, M. E. and Havens, I. (1947). Studies on immunity to asiatic cholera IV. The excretion of copro antibody in the guinea pig. J. Infect. Dis., **81**, 261

Cooper, M. D. and Lawton, A. R. (1973). The mammalian "bursa equivalent". Contemp. Topics. Immunobiol., **1**, 49

Craig, S. W. and Cebra, J. J. (1971). Peyer's patches: an enriched source of precursors for IgA producing immunocytes in the rabbit. J. Exp. Med., **134**, 188

Davies, A. (1922). Serological properties of dysentery stools. Lancet, **ii**, 1009

Ferguson, A. and Parrott, D. M. V. (1972). The effect of antigen deprivation on thymus-dependent and thymus-independent lymphocytes in the small intestine of the mouse. Clin. Exp. Immunol., **12**, 477

Gowans, J. L. and Knight, E. J. (1964). The route of recirculation of lymphocytes in the rat. Proc. R. Soc. **B, 159**, 257

Griscelli, C., Vassalli, P. and McCluskey, R. T. (1969). The distribution of large dividing lymph node cells in syngeneic recipients after intravenous injection. J. Exp. Med., **130**, 1427

Guy-Grand, D., Griscelli, C. and Vassalli, P. (1974). The gut-associated lymphoid system: nature and properties of large dividing cells. Eur. J. Immunol., **4**, 435

Guy-Grand, D., Griscelli, C. and Vassalli, P. (1975). Peyer's patches, gut IgA plasma cells and thymic function: study in nude mice bearing thymic grafts. J. Immunol., **115**, 361

Hall, J. G. (1971). The lymph-borne cells of the immune response: a review. Scientific Basis of Medicine. Annual Reviews. pp.39-57. Athlone Press

Hall, J. G., Parry, D. M. and Smith, M. E. (1972). The distribution and differentiations of lymph-borne immunoblasts after intravenous injection into syngeneic recipients. Cell. Tissue Kinet., **5**, 269

Hall, J. G. and Smith, M. E. (1970). Homing of lymph-borne immunoblasts to the gut. Nature, **226**, 262

Halstead, T. E. and Hall, J. G. (1972). The homing of lymph-borne immunoblasts to the small gut of neonatal rats. Transplantation, **14**, 339

Heath, T. J., Lascelles, A. K. and Morris, B. (1962). The cells of sheep lymph. J. Anat., **96**, 397

Heremans, J. F. (1974). Immunoglobulin A. In: (M. Sela (ed.) The Antigens 2, pp.365. (New York and London: Academic Press)

Hopkins, J. and Hall, J. G. (1976). Selective entry of immunoblasts into gut from intestinal lymph. Nature, **259**, 308

McMaster, P. D. (1961). Antibody formation. In: (J. Brachet and A. E. Mirsky (eds.) The Cell **5**, pp.323—404. (New York and London: Academic Press)

Mandel, M. A. and Asofsky, R. (1968). Studies on thoracic duct lymphocytes in mice. J. Immunol., **100**, 363

Miller, J. F. A. P. (1963). Origins of immunological competence. Br. Med. Bull., **19**, 214

Moore, A. R. and Hall, J. G. (1972). Evidence for a primary association between lymphocytes and the small gut. Nature, **239**, 161

Ogra, P. L. and Karzon, D. T. (1969). Distribution of polio virus antibody in serum, nasopharynx and alimentary tract following segmental immunization of lower alimentary tract with polio vaccine. J. Immunol., **102**, 1423

Parrott, D. M. V., de Sousa, M. A. and East, J. (1966). Thymus dependent areas in the lymphoid organs of neonatally thymectomized mice. J. Exp. Med., **123**, 191

Pearson, L. D., Simpson-Morgan, M. W. and Morris, B. (1976). Lymphopoesis and lymphocyte recirculation in the sheep fetus. J. Exp. Med., **143**, 167

Peyer, J. C. (1677). Exercitatio anat. de glandulis intestinorum earumque usu et affectionibus. Cited by Garrison, F. H. (1929). An Introduction to the History of Medicine. 4th Edition.

Pierce, A. E. (1959). Specific antibodies at mucous surfaces. Vet. Revs. Annots., **5**, 17

Pierce, N. F. and Gowans, J. L. (1975). Cellular kinetics of the intestinal immune response to cholera toxoid in rats. J. Exp. Med., **142**, 1550

Porter, P., Noakes, D E. and Allen, W. D. (1970). Intestinal secretion of immunoglobulins and antibodies to E. coli in the pig. Immunology, **18**, 909

Scollay, R. G., Hall, J. G. and Orlans, E. (1976). Studies on the lymphocytes of sheep. II. Some properties of cells in various compartments of the recirculating lymphocyte pool. Eur. J. Immunol., **6**, 121

Scollay, R. G., Hopkins, J. and Hall, J. G. (1976). Possible role of surface Ig in non-random recirculation of small lymphocytes. Nature, **260**, 528

Smith, J. B., McIntosh, G. H. and Morris, B. (1970). The traffic of cells through tissues: a study of peripheral lymph in sheep. J. Anat., **107**, 87

de Sousa, M. A. (1973). Ecology of thymus dependency. Contemp. Top. Immunobiol., **2**, 119

Sprent, J. (1976). Fate of H2-activated T-lymphocytes in syngeneic hosts. Cell. Immunol., **21**, 278

Tourville, D. R., Adler, R. H., Bienenstock, J. and Tomasi, T. B. (1969). The human secretory globulin system. Immunohistological localization of γA, secretory piece and lactoferrin in normal human tissues. J. Exp. Med., **129**, 411

POSTSCRIPT

Since I wrote this paper, some points have become clearer. The migratory behaviour of GALT derived cells in lambs in utero, and the characteristics of cells in the peripheral lymph of the intestine have been published (Hall et al., 1977). More important, though, have been the findings that bile is a rich source of secretory IgA (Lemaitre-Coelho et al., 1977) and that this immunoglobulin is transported rapidly and actively by the hepatocytes from blood to bile (Orlans et al., 1978). These findings apply directly only to rodents but there is evidence already that a similar phenomenon occurs in most mammals, including man, even though there may be considerable differences in detail between species. There can be little doubt that biliary IgA and associated glycoproteins will become factors of the first importance in any future consideration of antigen absorbtion by the gut.

References

Hall, J. G., Hopkins, J. and Orlans, E. (1977). Studies on the lymphocytes of sheep. III Destination of lymph-borne immunoblasts in relation to their tissue of origin. Eur. J. Immunol., **7**, 30

Lemaître-Coelho, I., Jackson, G. D. F. and Vaerman, J. P. (1977). Rat bile as a convenient source of IgA and free secretory component. Eur. J. Immunol., **8**, 588

Orlans, E., Peppard, J., Reynolds, J. and Hall, J. G. (1978). Rapid active transport of immunoglobulin A from blood to bile. J. Exp. Med., **147**, 588

22
Summing up

J. L. GOWANS

The traditional duty of a Chairman in summing up a Conference is to ensure that he mentions each of the speakers in turn and compliments them on their contribution. I don't propose to do this on the present occasion as I do not think that any of the contributors needs a boost to his amour propre and I will simply say that the standard of presentation has been very high and that it has been a very interesting meeting.

I should like to mention one or two topics on gut immunity which have interested me particularly. I shall not be commenting on the first five papers in this symposium which dealt with the absorption of macromolecules by very young animals and where several speakers dealt with the problem of the nature and specificity of receptors in the gut. This is a topic which is of course dear to the hearts of this laboratory but it is one which is new to me and I have nothing to add to what has already been said.

We ourselves have been interested in the mechanism by which intestinal immunity is generated in rats. It is a striking observation that the lamina propria of the intestine of normal rats, and of many other mammalian species, contains numerous cells which are secreting IgA into the intestinal lumen. The obvious question to ask is what these IgA molecules are antibodies against? I came to this meeting thinking that the small gut was relatively sterile but we were told by Dr. Lee this is not true, certainly for the lower half of the small intestine. So possibly plasma cells in the gut are making antibodies against bacterial antigens. However, in comparison with the small intestine the bacterial load in the large intestine is enormous but there are not a commensurately larger number of IgA secreting cells in the large gut. A second possibility to account for the antibody producing cells in the small intestine, which has been aired at this meeting, is that the antibodies are directed against dietary proteins which might otherwise be absorbed unchanged into the circulation. This notion stems partly from a claim that a first dose of antigen by mouth changes the animal in some way so that a second dose is not absorbed, the idea being that antibodies generated by the priming dose combine with the second dose and prevent its absorption. A dramatic observation which is new to me is that even in adult animals a large proportion of certain proteins can be absorbed and detected in immunogenic form in the body of the animal. Thus Dr. Hemmings has shown that up to 20% of a dose of either Ferritin or heterologous IgG after administration by the gut can be recovered in the carcase of the animal. Thus, it seems reasonable to suppose that immunological mechanisms might prevent the continual ingress of foreign protein and that such a mechanism is revealed when a protein new to the animal is presented to the intestinal epithelium.

There seems to be some dispute about whether the second of two doses of antigen given into the gut can elicit a secondary antibody response. Employing as antigen either sheep erythrocytes or a curious organism isolated from a concrete pipe in Tasmania it was claimed that the second dose of antigen by mouth did not result in a response larger than that given by the first. However, another paper alleged that the serum antibody titre in an animal given diphtheria toxoid into the intestine was raised after the second dose of antigen. I can add a little to this debate by quoting some results that Dr. Pierce and I obtained in rats immunized with cholera toxoid (1). We were interested in defining the best conditions for raising intestinal immunity to this antigen and we discovered that a brisk secondary response could be obtained if the regime of immunization was accurately defined. If a single dose of toxoid was given intraperitoneally very few specific antibody forming cells appeared in the lamina propria of the intestine but some IgC antibody appeared in the blood. However, following challenge with antigen, given either in the drinking water or by direct injection into the lumen of the gut, a secondary response was detected by two methods. First, it was found that during the week after challenge considerable numbers of specific antitoxin containing cells (ACC) accumulated in the lamina propria of the small gut and the antibody they contained was predominantly IgA. Second, we showed that after the primed animal was challenged via the gut a surge of ACC appeared rapidly in the thoracic duct lymph and that again the antibody was almost exclusively of the class, IgA. I think these two kinds of measurements justify the conclusion that the gut secretory antibody system was mounting a secondary immune response. In order to obtain such a response it was necessary to challenge the animal by way of the gut; intraperitoneal priming followed by intraperitoneal boosting gave substantial levels of antibody in the blood but did not result in the accumulation of ACC in the lamina propria. Recent studies have suggested that the antibody forming cells which appear in the lymph are derived from the Peyer's patches (2) which are organs attracting a great deal of interest at the moment. The role of Peyer's patches in generating IgA secreting cells considerably weakens earlier claims that they might be part of a central lymphoid mass, analogous to the bursa of Fabricius in birds.

The link between the two measurements of the secondary response which I have just mentioned is obviously that the cells which are fired off into the lymph as a result of intestinal challenge pass into the blood and then migrate into the lamina propria to provide the IgA secreting cells. This conclusion is supported by the observation that the number of ACC which accumulated in the lamina propria after challenge was dramatically reduced in animals with a thoracic duct fistula draining to the exterior. Direct evidence for the migration of these cells comes from transfusion studies in which radiolabelled large lymphocytes from the thoracic duct were identified in the lamina propria of recipient animals carrying both the radioactive label and internal IgA.

The problem which has been left unsolved by these experiments, and which has been touched upon in the present symposium, is the mechanism by which the circulating large lymphocytes are attracted into the lamina propria. There is conflicting evidence about the influence of antigen on the homing of these cells although, on general grounds, antigen might be thought to be the strongest candidate since it would be sensible to deliver the antibody-producing cells to the site where antigen needs to be neutralized. Experiments described to us today have shown that antigen introduced into isolated loops of gut results in the production of antibody locally in the loop. On the other hand, transfusion experiments have suggested that large lymphocytes home randomly to the whole small intestine and, indeed, will home into intestine derived from embryonic or neonatal animals where the gut is presumably sterile (3, 4). I do not yet know how these two sets of observations can be reconciled. The intestine seems to provide an intrinsic attraction for large lymphocytes and, in addition, antigen seems to have an important influence on the region of the gut into which they migrate (4). There have been suggestions that the first of these two phenomena might be explained by the presence of IgA on the surface of large lymphocytes and the presence of secretory component (which can combine with dimeric IgA) in the intestine. This suggestion is attractive because it is very easy to design experiments to test it, but for the moment we have too little information to make further speculation profitable.

In conclusion I am sure you would like me to say on your behalf what a splendid conference this has been. We have all enjoyed the hospitality of the University College of North Wales and of Dr. Hemmings personally. We have considered topics as disparate as brush borders and mental disease and if you have all benefited as much as I have from the range and vigour of the discussions then the conference must be judged as an outstanding success.

References

1. Pierce, N. F. and Gowans, J. L. (1975) J. Exp. Med., **142**, 1550
2. Craig, S. W. and Cebra, J. J. (1971) J. Exp. Med., **134**, 18
3. Parrott, D. M. V. and Ferguson, A. (1974) Immunology, **26**, 571
4. Halsted, T. E. and Hall, J. G. (1972) Transplantation, **14**, 339

Index